T0047383

Praise for *What Every V* *to Know About Fertility*

'Are you a woman wanting to avoid pregnancy and would prefer to use fertility awareness methods. Or to plan one? Or are you experiencing difficulties in conceiving? Are you a partner, or even family member or friend, of someone in that position? This book should be *essential reading* and is highly recommended. It is written with warmth, understanding and expertise by two long-standing professionals in this field. Authoritative, based on clear evidence, it is designed to be dipped into, or read cover to cover and will have something of interest for anybody. Authors Knight and Belfield have set out to write a guidebook that will reassure and answer just about every question you might have on the subject – and have succeeded.'

Suzie Hayman, agony aunt, relationship counsellor
and parenting practitioner

'In an age where pregnancy can now be a choice, women have never been in more need of authoritative yet supportive advice about that important decision. *What Every Woman Needs to Know about Fertility*, written by two experienced specialist health professionals meets that need, offering accurate information, focused insight and helpful guidance into both getting and not getting pregnant. The authors have effectively managed to inform and inspire their readers as they face (what I know from my work with clients who enter the battlefield of fertility) the huge challenge of conception or not. Essential reading for choosing the right reproductive options for you.'

Susan Quilliam, relationship advice columnist,
author of (the revised) The Joy of Sex

'What an empowering read! It gives every woman who is (or is thinking of being) sexually active the calm and detailed facts to make effective decisions about her fertility – and is essential reading for partners, too.'

Deidre Sanders MBE, agony aunt on ITV's 'This Morning',
long-time editor of The Sun's 'Dear Deidre' problem page

'This highly informative yet easy-to-read book exploring fertility awareness will guide potential users through the complexities of managing their birth control without the need for hormones or barrier methods. Being able to understand how our bodies work is explained with the aid of informative images and charts. This book will also be invaluable for those planning pregnancies highlighting

the most fertile days and ensuring good preconception advice.
I think this book will also be a welcomed addition to the bookshelf of every healthcare professional working in the field of contraception and reproductive health, along with those in primary care and gynaecology.'

Dr Diana Mansour, Consultant in Community Gynaecology, Newcastle-upon-Tyne

'A beautifully clear, detailed and up-to-date account of fertility awareness. This is the go-to book for those wanting either to avoid or achieve pregnancy.'

Prof Sam Rowlands, Visiting Professor, Department of Medical Science and Public Health, Bournemouth University

'This is the resource I wish I'd had to help discuss fertility with everyone – users, colleagues and students.'

Shelley Raine, Nurse Specialist in Contraception, Hampshire

'A great resource for women, their partners and health professionals wanting clear accurate information about fertility awareness for both avoiding and planning pregnancy.'

Prof Jill Shawe, Professor Maternal and Family Health, University of Plymouth

'In this comprehensive, evidence-based and highly user-friendly book, the authors have confirmed the importance of fertility education and choice through balanced, honest information that corrects the many inaccuracies fuelled by social media.'

John Guillebaud, Emeritus Professor of Family Planning and Reproductive Health, University College, London

What Every Woman Needs to Know About Fertility

What Every Woman Needs to Know About Fertility

Your Guide to Fertility Awareness to Plan or Avoid Pregnancy

JANE KNIGHT AND TONI BELFIELD

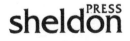

First published by Sheldon Press in 2023
An imprint of John Murray Press

1

Copyright © Jane Knight and Toni Belfield 2023

The right of Jane Knight and Toni Belfield to be identified as the Authors of the Work has been asserted by them in accordance with the Copyright, Designs and Patents Act 1988.

All rights reserved. No part of this publication may be reproduced, stored in a retrieval system, or transmitted, in any form or by any means without the prior written permission of the publisher, nor be otherwise circulated in any form of binding or cover other than that in which it is published and without a similar condition being imposed on the subsequent purchaser.

This book is for information or educational purposes only and is not intended to act as a substitute for medical advice or treatment. Any person with a condition requiring medical attention should consult a qualified medical practitioner or suitable therapist.

A CIP catalogue record for this title is available from the British Library

Trade Paperback ISBN 9781399814591
eBook ISBN 9781399814607

Typeset by KnowledgeWorks Global Ltd.

Printed and bound in Great Britain by Clays Ltd, Elcograf S.p.A.

John Murray Press policy is to use papers that are natural, renewable and recyclable products and made from wood grown in sustainable forests. The logging and manufacturing processes are expected to conform to the environmental regulations of the country of origin.

John Murray Press
Carmelite House
50 Victoria Embankment
London EC4Y 0DZ

Nicholas Brealey Publishing
Hachette Book Group
Market Place, Center 53, State Street
Boston, MA 02109, USA

www.sheldonpress.co.uk
John Murray Press, part of Hodder & Stoughton Limited
An Hachette UK company

Contents

List of figures

Acknowledgements

Thank you to all the women we have spoken with over the years. This book is for you.

Thank you to our peer reviewers:

- Prof Sam Rowlands – Visiting Professor, Department of Medical Science and Public Health, Bournemouth University
- Dr Diana Mansour – Consultant in Community Gynaecology, Newcastle
- Prof Jill Shawe – Professor Maternal and Family Health, University of Plymouth
- Shelley Raine – Nurse Specialist in Contraception, Hampshire
- Sue Everett – Associate Professor and Senior Teaching Fellow, Department of Nursing, Midwifery, Faculty of Health, Social Care and Education, Middlesex University.

Thank you to practitioners on the FertilityUK network for demonstrating the demand for this book and for their encouragement and support while writing.

Thank you to Dr Cecilia Pyper for her permission to use some of the lovely physiology images and to Pia Gill at Burnt Peach Design for her work on the book's helpful images and charts.

Images and permissions

Artwork by Burnt Peach Design.

Figures 2.1, 2.6, 2.8, 3.2, 3.3–3.13 and 4.1/Appendix: Blank chart for planning preganancy with instructions for use: copyright © Jane Knight, 2016. Adapted from *The Complete Guide to Fertility Awareness*, Jane Knight, Routledge 2017.

Figures 2.2, 2.3, 2.4, 2.5, 3.1, 3.14: copyright © Dr Cecilia Pyper and Jane Knight 2016. Produced in collaboration with FertilityUK and the Institute for Reproductive Health, Georgetown University. Adapted from *The Complete Guide to Fertility Awareness*, Jane Knight, Routledge 2017.

Figure 2.7 adapted from Wilcox, A. J., Weinberg, C. R. and Baird D. D., Dec 1995, Timing of sexual intercourse in relation to ovulation. *New England Journal of Medicine* 333(23): 1517–21.

Disclaimer

The information contained in this book is based on evidence and medical opinion at the time of publication. Care has been taken to ensure that the information given is accurate and up-to-date. Medical knowledge and practice changes as new information becomes available necessitating changes in treatment, drugs or practice. This book aims to improve understanding of fertility awareness and provide detail of the methods to plan or avoid pregnancy. However, to use fertility awareness methods effectively, it is strongly recommended that you have supplementary teaching and ongoing support from an accredited practitioner – this is particularly important if you wish to avoid pregnancy.

About this book

Knowledge about fertility and reproductive health is generally lacking across all age groups. Surveys show that this is even the case among women who have painstakingly trawled through books and the Internet to try to improve their understanding of fertility, conception and pregnancy. Misinformation about the menstrual cycle and the fertile time commonly results in unintended pregnancies for those trying to avoid pregnancy and fertility delays for those trying to conceive. There is also widespread confusion about the impact of age on fertility. A woman's fertility actually starts to decline in her late twenties with a more rapid decline by her mid-thirties. So, for some women, delaying childbearing until their mid-thirties could mean they have 'left it too late'. In the UK, about one in five couples remain childless – some by choice, others by circumstance. Fertility has been described as a 'gift with an expiry date'.

The information in this book will help you to take control of your fertility and make informed choices at all stages of your reproductive life. It will alert you to signs and symptoms which will help you understand your body better and could indicate gynaecological problems, for example polycystic ovaries or endometriosis, and give you clear red flags for signs requiring urgent medical advice. The book will help you to consider whether and when you might want to start a family, prepare for pregnancy, modify your lifestyle and boost your chances of conception. The text is guided by the best objective scientific evidence from organizations such as the Royal College of Obstetricians and Gynaecologists (RCOG), the Faculty of Sexual and Reproductive Healthcare (FSRH) and the National Institute for Health and Care Excellence (NICE). Each section clearly signposts you to the most authoritative and relevant sources of further information. Contact details for all relevant organizations are listed in the resources section at the back of the book.

If you are looking for a more natural method of contraception, you will learn how to accurately identify the fertile time so that you can either abstain from intercourse or use a barrier method during the fertile time. It is strongly recommended that you are taught by an experienced practitioner and that you have their ongoing support, but this practical guide will help to boost your confidence in the method by providing a vital source of written information with a step-by-step approach to interpreting your charts and clear guidelines to back up the teaching.

There is no 'right' way to read this book – you can choose to read it from cover to cover and then go back to the most relevant sections, or you may prefer to dip in and out. At the back of the book, you will find a handy glossary of terms. Chapter 1 gives an overview of fertility awareness and its relevance at different life stages. Chapter 2 and Chapter 3 are essential reading – they are fundamental to your understanding of fertility – so these are not to be missed. You can then go straight to the chapter that best suits your situation. If you are planning pregnancy, you can jump straight to Chapter 8. For anyone experiencing delays in conceiving, Chapter 9 looks at the causes of infertility, when to seek further tests and investigations and the available treatments. It also addresses the importance of age on fertility, the realistic chances of pregnancy for older women and the increasing use of assisted conception including donated eggs.

If you are avoiding pregnancy, make sure you read Chapter 4 thoroughly. Then, if appropriate, you can skip to the most relevant chapter for your circumstances – whether you are wanting to change your method of contraception, such as stopping hormonal contraception, breastfeeding or approaching the menopause. At the end of the book, you will find blank charts to record your temperature and other indicators. These can also be downloaded from the FertilityUK website – see teaching organizations in the Resources section.

Throughout this book we use Celsius (also known as centigrade) when referring to temperature measurement. Over the last 50-plus years, the vast majority of countries have switched from the imperial to the metric system – the main exception being the USA which still uses the Fahrenheit scale. Ideally, to avoid any errors, you should use a Celsius digital thermometer, but if this is not possible you can use a Fahrenheit thermometer. A Fahrenheit scale is included on the blank chart at the back of the book showing 0.1 degrees Celsius equivalent to 0.2 degrees Fahrenheit. So, when the text refers to the third high temperature being at least 0.2 degrees Celsius higher, this will be 0.4 degrees Fahrenheit higher. Some thermometers show both temperature scales. The important thing is to be consistent. If you want to switch, then do so at the start of a new cycle.

One might reasonably ask why women still need to bother learning about their menstrual cycle when there are over 1,000 fertility apps on the market claiming to know when a woman is ovulating or might expect her next period. Undoubtedly, female technology (sometimes referred to as femtech) is the way things are going; however, these products are unregulated and have serious limitations including concerns about false or confusing claims for their effectiveness. There are also privacy issues with data sharing. If you want to use an app, it is vital that you really understand how it works and you use the technology intelligently – this essentially means that you need to understand your fertility and recognize how external factors (such as alcohol, illness, disturbed sleep or stress) impact on your menstrual cycles. Too many women are caught out by blindly trusting their app. It is not enough to expect an app alone to deliver – however costly or well it is marketed.

What Every Woman Needs to Know about Fertility, written by two highly experienced practitioners – a specialist fertility nurse and a specialist in sexual and reproductive health information – provides a single authoritative source of information that you can trust. Here we talk about women and women's reproductive health, and men and men's reproductive health. We recognize that how you choose to identify yourself is a personal choice and that it is important to acknowledge that everyone has the right to access good reproductive health information and services and that care should be appropriate, sensitive and inclusive. The information and facts in this book relate to people whose gender identity is the same as the sex determined at conception and assigned at birth. We use the word 'woman' (and the pronouns 'she' and 'her') to describe individuals whose sex assigned at birth was female (whether they identify as female, male or non-binary), and 'man' ('he' and 'him') to describe individuals whose sex assigned at birth was male whether they identify as male, female or non-binary.

1

Fertility awareness

Fertility awareness: an essential education for all

Some of the most common things women say once they become aware of their fertility are: 'I wish I had known earlier', 'Why didn't we learn this at school?' or 'We are told about contraception, but never about how our bodies work or how to get pregnant'. This is why fertility awareness is such an essential part of education for all of us whatever our gender or sexual orientation. Women and men need to know about reproduction and understand how their bodies work. Fertility awareness helps young people to understand bodily changes associated with puberty and to value their fertility. Young women need to know about the normal variations in the menstrual cycle and learn to distinguish between normal and abnormal vaginal secretions. Many find it fascinating to track their periods, notice how cycles can be affected by stress or illness and how hormonal changes can affect mood. Fertility awareness gives young women confidence in their ability to conceive and, importantly, a realization of the need to protect against sexually transmitted infections and unintended pregnancies. Young people need to consider whether and when they might want to have children and to understand that fertility declines with age, recognizing that the most fertile years of a woman's reproductive life are between 18 and 30 years.

Fertility awareness methods (FAMs): part of contraceptive choice

Fertility awareness knowledge is fundamental to an understanding of how different contraceptive methods work, how they interrupt fertility to prevent pregnancy and how fertility returns after stopping the method. Contraceptive needs change at different life stages. Most young people have a crucial need to avoid pregnancy while completing their education and settling into a career or work environment; there may then be a more

1

relaxed approach to contraception once they are settled in the 'right' relationship – this is a common time for women to seek out a more natural method of contraception. It can, however, be notoriously difficult to find accurate, objective information about fertility awareness methods (FAMs). Information is often confusing as there is an abundance of apps and different 'methods' with a whole variety of names, each claiming to be the most 'advanced'. What is needed are straightforward facts based on the best scientific evidence and an understanding of how this can be applied to suit personal circumstances. Understanding the signs and symptoms of fertility during the menstrual cycle allows you to take control of your fertility – to plan or avoid pregnancy.

Fertility awareness to plan pregnancy

Fertility awareness knowledge can help to boost your chances of pregnancy and optimize preconception care. Understanding the variation in the length of your menstrual cycles and the changes in the vaginal secretions which indicate high fertility helps you to improve sex timing. If you have been having frequent sexual intercourse, but have not conceived after about six months, seek medical advice. About one in seven heterosexual couples face difficulties conceiving.

Fertility awareness methods to avoid pregnancy

Fertility awareness methods include all family planning methods that are based on identifying the fertile time. If you are using FAMs to avoid pregnancy, there are a number of days in the menstrual cycle when unprotected sex could result in pregnancy. So, you and your partner will have to consider how to have protected sex during the fertile time: you can either use barrier methods (condoms or a diaphragm) or abstain from intercourse – the choice is yours. Strictly speaking, natural family planning (NFP) implies abstinence during the fertile time; if you use barrier methods, this is usually referred to as FAMs with barriers or simply FAMs.

The evolution of modern fertility awareness methods

It is helpful to have an idea of how fertility awareness methods have evolved over the last century. In 1929, Kyusaku Ogino (in Japan) and

Hermann Knaus (in Austria) independently established that ovulation occurs at a fixed time (about 10–16 days) *before* the next period – this led to the development of the calendar/rhythm method. Provided women had regular cycles, this worked pretty well compared with using no method, but we now know that sperm can survive considerably longer than thought at that time. By the 1950s, the science showed a slight but detectable rise in body temperature after ovulation. J. G. H. Holt (a Dutch gynaecologist) and John Marshall (a British neurologist) developed this into a practical method – the temperature method. Temperature as a single indicator was a highly effective method for avoiding pregnancy once ovulation had been confirmed, but there was limited time for intercourse which caused difficulties (and many unintended pregnancies). Gynaecologists were increasingly researching the changes in the cervix and its secretions. In the 1960s, two Australian doctors (John and Evelyn Billings) developed the ovulation method, which is still widely used today. Each fertility indicator has its own merits, but also its limitations – research now clearly shows that using a combination of indicators gives the most effective method for avoiding pregnancy.

Fertility awareness methods in today's world

When motivated couples wanting to avoid pregnancy are taught by accredited practitioners to use a combination of fertility signs correctly and consistently, modern FAMs are up to 99 per cent effective – that is one woman in 100 would get pregnant over the course of one year. Without proper instruction and support, however, many more pregnancies will result – this is definitely not a DIY method. For a list of FAM practitioners, see Resources.

Who uses fertility awareness methods?

Many women seek out FAMs because they want to use something that is natural or are struggling to find a contraceptive method that suits them. Moving from a method that requires less thought to one where you will be making decisions about your fertility on a day-to-day basis requires commitment by you and the support of your partner. You do not need to have regular menstrual cycles to use FAMs, but it can be more difficult to learn (and more restrictive) if your cycles are irregular and at times of hormonal change. Women who are coming off hormonal methods may have several months of cycle disturbance, making it more challenging to find the infertile (safe) time. Women who are fully breastfeeding can enjoy the time of natural infertility when spacing their babies and learn to watch for returning fertility during weaning. Women who are approaching the menopause can observe their declining fertility, understand their menopausal symptoms and feel reassured when their fertility has ceased. FAMs may not be suitable for some women – for example those who have a medical condition which could make pregnancy a high risk for themselves or those taking prescribed drugs which could cause congenital abnormalities.

Advantages and disadvantages of FAMs

The following list contains well-recognized advantages and disadvantages of FAMs, but this is very personal – every individual will find their own unique benefits and challenges.

Advantages

- Helps you to know and understand your body
- Improves awareness of reproductive and sexual health
- Gives an early warning of signs which require medical advice
- No chemical substances or physical devices
- Free from side effects
- No adverse effects on future fertility
- Effective when well taught and used by motivated couples
- Encourages shared responsibility and communication between partners
- Puts couples in control of their fertility – for planning and avoiding pregnancy
- Acceptable to those with ethical, cultural or religious concerns
- Can be used in combination with barrier methods
- Helps to optimize intercourse timing to conceive
- Improves chances of conception for subfertile couples.
- Low cost for methods based on self-observation

Disadvantages

- Takes time to learn (three to six cycles)
- Some women find charting cumbersome
- Requires the co-operation and commitment of both partners
- Requires modification to patterns of sexual activity
- Some couples have difficulties with abstinence
- More difficult at times of stress or hormonal change
- No protection against sexually transmitted infections
- High risk of pregnancy with imperfect use and risk-taking
- May increase fear of unintended pregnancy, particularly during the learning phase
- High-quality teaching services may not be easily accessible
- Fertility monitoring devices can be prohibitively expensive
- Most apps and devices have not been tested in independent clinical trials
- Limited regulation of fertility apps

2

Understanding fertility and conception

Understanding how your body works and knowing about the male and female reproductive systems – what they are and what they do – will help you know more about your fertility and your ability to conceive and have children. Fertility awareness involves being able to identify the signs and symptoms of fertility during the menstrual cycle. It is important to say that every woman is different and that, although the principles are the same, no two bodies or menstrual cycles are the same. Each woman is an individual and learning more about your own body and how it works will give you confidence physically and emotionally.

Women's bodies

The reproductive system in women is made up of external and internal organs. They are found in the lower abdomen, the part of the body below the umbilicus (tummy/belly button). This area is referred to as the pelvic area.

The external organs, known collectively as the vulva, are:

- the vaginal entrance
- the urethral opening (tube from the bladder through which you urinate)
- the labia
- the clitoris.

The woman's external reproductive organs (genitals) (Figure 2.1) are all visible; they vary in size and appearance from one woman to another. The pubic mound (mons pubis) is a soft, fatty pad that covers and protects the pubic bone. It is naturally covered with pubic hair. The labia consist of two fleshy lips – the labia majora (outer lips) and the labia minora (inner lips). These lips protect the vagina and they

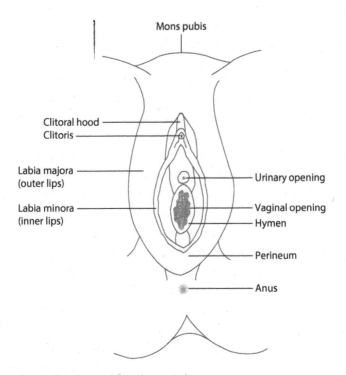

Mons pubis

Clitoral hood

Clitoris

Labia majora
(outer lips)

Labia minora
(inner lips)

Urinary opening

Vaginal opening

Hymen

Perineum

Anus

Figure 2.1 External female genitals

contain sensitive nerve endings. During sexual arousal and intercourse these lips become engorged with blood and become moist to help penetration of the penis. The external part of the clitoris is found towards the front of the vulva. It is made up of highly sensitive erectile tissue and is the female equivalent of the male glans penis. When stimulated during sexual activity this leads to sexual arousal and orgasm. The hymen is a thin layer of soft skin that surrounds or partially covers the vaginal opening. This easily becomes stretched and opened with the use of tampons, physical exercise and intercourse. Importantly, the physical state of the hymen is not an indicator of a woman's virginity or sexual experience. The area between the external organs and the anus (excretory opening or back passage) is known as the perineum.

⚠ Female genital mutilation (FGM)

In some countries, women are subjected to female 'circumcision' for religious, cultural or traditional reasons. Whereas in men, circumcision involves simple surgical removal of the foreskin (which covers the head of the penis) usually for medical reasons and in some instances for tradition, as in, for example, Judaism; in women, 'circumcision' involves genital cutting which results in partial or total removal of the external female genitals or other injury to the female genital organs for non-medical reasons – this is female genital mutilation (FGM). Female genital mutilation is extremely harmful and can result in short- and long-term damage to the reproductive organs. It can cause infection and often results in complications during pregnancy and childbirth, sexual dysfunction and menstrual problems.

If you have had FGM, ask your GP for referral to a specialist NHS gynaecologist to discuss your health needs. Alternatively, you can find your local FGM support clinic through the NHS website. Also see Resources for the organization Forward. Female genital mutilation, virginity testing and hymenoplasty (where the hymen is surgically reconstructed) are illegal in the UK.

The internal reproductive organs (Figure 2.2) are:

- the ovaries
- the fallopian tubes
- the uterus (womb)
- the cervix
- the vagina.

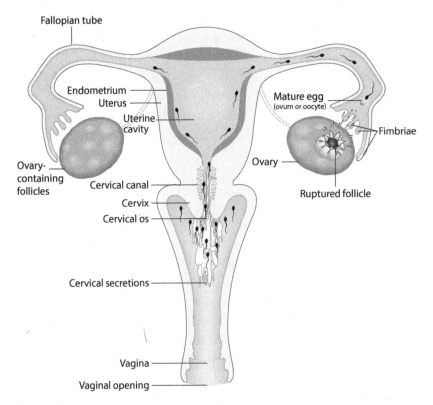

Figure 2.2 Female reproductive organs
© Pyper & Knight, FertilityUK 2016

Ovaries

Women have two ovaries – one on each side of the uterus. They are the size and shape of almonds and they produce eggs (ova/oocytes) in structures called follicles. The ovaries also produce two female sex hormones – estrogen and progesterone. Each egg contains chromosomes (genes that determine our sex and what we look like).

When a baby girl is born, she is born with all the eggs she needs for her lifetime. At birth, there are around 1–2 million immature (not yet developed) eggs in her ovaries, but by puberty there are only about 100,000 left. Most of these eggs will never be released; they are absorbed naturally by the ovaries. Once a woman starts having periods (menarche) and an established menstrual cycle, the ovaries select up to 20 resting follicles to start to grow and mature. One follicle becomes dominant and releases its mature egg at ovulation while the other eggs degenerate. During her reproductive years, some 300–400 eggs will mature and be released at ovulation.

As a woman gets older, the quality and quantity of her eggs decline, which affects her chances of becoming pregnant, carrying a pregnancy and having a healthy baby. For this reason, the ideal time biologically to become pregnant and have a baby is between the ages of 18 and 30.

Fast facts

- The female sex hormones estrogen and progesterone are responsible for female characteristics such as body shape, developing breasts, periods and controlling the menstrual cycle.
- The ovaries contain about 1–2 million immature eggs at birth.
- During a woman's reproductive life only about 300–400 eggs will actually be released at ovulation.
- As a woman gets older (over 35) the number and quality of her eggs decline, making conception more difficult, and miscarriage more common.
- Being 'on the pill' (or using any hormonal contraception that prevents ovulation) doesn't 'conserve' eggs. Having fertility treatment (such as IVF) doesn't use them up.
- An egg is the largest cell in the human body but still less than one-eighth of the size of a grain of sand and invisible to the naked eye.
- An egg only survives for up to 24 hours, but allowance is made in case a second egg is released (as with non-identical twins), increasing potential total egg survival time to 48 hours.

Fallopian tubes

The two fallopian tubes are found one on each side of the uterus, near the ovaries. A fringe of tissue (fimbriae) at the funnel-like end of the fallopian tube picks up the egg released by the ovary and helps move the egg along towards the uterus. Each tube is about 10 cm long. The inside of the tube is very delicate, the narrowest part being about 1 mm in diameter. The tubes are lined with microscopic hairs (cilia); these can easily be damaged or blocked by infections such as chlamydia, or a burst appendix. Thrush (yeast infection) does not cause blocked tubes.

Uterus

The uterus (womb) is about the size and shape of an upside-down pear. It is hollow, very stretchy and made of muscle. This is where the baby develops when a woman becomes pregnant. The uterus can stretch to hold a baby and shrink back more or less to its pre-pregnancy size after the baby is born. The lining of the uterus (endometrium) nourishes the newly fertilized egg and supports the development of the placenta and its umbilical cord – the tube that connects the baby to the mother during pregnancy providing vital nourishment and removing waste products.

The uterus is positioned in the pelvic cavity between the bladder and the rectum. In most women, it lies at an angle slightly tipped towards the pubic bone at right angles to the vagina. This is known as an anteverted anteflexed uterus. It is designed to be in a good position for intercourse and childbirth. About one in five women have a retroverted uterus; this means instead of being at right angles to the vagina, the uterus tips slightly backwards (towards the small of the back). This is often discovered when having cervical screening and usually causes no problems. Women using fertility awareness methods will notice the position of the cervix and may find out this way.

Cervix

This is the lower part of the uterus, which projects slightly into the vagina. The cervical canal links the cavity of the uterus with the vagina. The cervical opening into the vagina is known as the external cervical os. The cells lining the cervical canal produce secretions (cervical mucus). These secretions are produced continuously but alter in texture and quantity during a woman's menstrual cycle (and are altered in women using hormonal contraceptive methods). Learning to identify these changes can help identify the fertile and infertile times in the cycle. Around the time of ovulation – when a woman is in her fertile time – the cervical secretions change from being thick, sticky and creamy in colour to being thinner, wetter, clearer and stretchy – like raw egg white. These changes allow sperm to pass more easily through the cervical canal and reach the egg.

The cervix is important in protecting the internal reproductive system from infection. When a woman becomes pregnant, the cells lining the cervical canal produce a very thick plug of mucus to protect the developing baby. During labour and delivery, the cervix opens (dilates) to allow the baby to be born. After pregnancy, it returns to its normal size, shape and function.

Vagina

The vagina is a muscular, elastic canal about 7–10 cm long that leads from the cervix to the vaginal opening. It has an inner layer of mucus membrane forming soft folds (known as rugae). The vagina tilts upward and towards the small of the back. The muscular walls lie closely together, except during sexual arousal when it expands to hold a penis or sex toy. Like the uterus, the vaginal walls are very stretchy and strong, enabling it to hold a tampon, stretch around an erect penis during sex or a baby during delivery. The pelvic floor muscles lie at the lower end of the vagina and around the anus. A woman can learn to identify these muscles by squeezing the muscles – felt by stopping and starting urine flow. The strength or tone of these muscles is important: some women find that these muscles are weakened after vaginal delivery during childbirth and around the time of the menopause. Pelvic floor exercises (known as Kegel exercises) strengthen these muscles which helps to improve bladder control and can help with intercourse.

During a woman's reproductive life, the vagina is kept moist by vaginal and cervical secretions. These secretions change in amount and composition during the menstrual cycle. They are important in keeping the vagina, cervix and uterus healthy and free from infection. For most of the menstrual cycle the secretions are slightly acidic and harmful to sperm; however, during a woman's fertile time, the cervical secretions become more alkaline and this has a neutralizing effect, protecting the sperm and allowing sperm survival.

Small pea-sized glands (Bartholin's glands) situated near the entrance to the vagina produce a colourless fluid (arousal fluid) in response to sexual stimulation. This provides vaginal lubrication in preparation for intercourse. The increased blood flow to vaginal tissues during sexual excitement also causes secretion of more fluids through the vaginal walls.

Your healthy vagina

A healthy vagina provides a suitable environment for friendly lactic-acid-producing bacteria, which protect against infection and provide a unique self-cleansing mechanism; however, some things may disturb the delicate pH (acidity or alkalinity) balance of your vagina.

- Avoid wearing tight, restrictive or synthetic clothing, such as nylon underwear, leggings, Lycra shorts, and tight jeans or trousers for long periods of time.
- Limit your use of tampons to days of moderate to heavy flow and use the minimal absorbency.
- Try to wear pads on lighter flow days, or days of spotting.
- Thongs can be very drying and increase your risk of thrush and cystitis.
- Make sure your vagina is well lubricated – either naturally or by using additional vaginal lubricant before sexual intercourse.
- Wash and wipe your genital area from front to back.

Most importantly, men and women should *always* avoid genital sprays, douches and deodorants, and any other irritants such as disinfectants and antiseptics. These can damage delicate tissues and can be dangerous. These are widely advertised as good perfumed things to use; they are not.

If you are prescribed any antibiotics, remind your doctor if you tend to get thrush and ask for some treatment for thrush at the same time (see Chapter 8). Some medications alter the effectiveness of hormonal contraceptive methods, so always ask about this if these are prescribed.

Breasts

Breasts contain milk glands, lymph nodes (immune centres) and fat. Pectoral muscles lie behind the breasts. Breasts change considerably throughout a woman's reproductive life, changing during each menstrual cycle in readiness for a possible pregnancy and enlarging during pregnancy as a result of milk production for breastfeeding.

Some women notice breast tenderness or tingling around the time of ovulation. Breasts may feel fuller, heavier and more painful in the second part of the menstrual cycle due to fluid retention caused by higher amounts of progesterone. Some women find they go up a bra cup-size in the time leading up to a period. These changes are important to recognize and understand why they happen, but they do not accurately reflect your fertile time.

ⓘ Breast awareness

Breasts come in all shapes and sizes and this is normal. Make sure that you are breast aware – this means being aware of the normal shape, size and consistency of your breast tissue remembering that it extends up into the armpit. Many women have quite lumpy breasts before a period. Any single lumps or different changes should be reported to your doctor immediately, but be reassured that about 90 per cent of breast lumps are not cancerous. Breast Cancer Now provides important information on breast awareness, benign (non-malignant) breast disease and all aspects of breast cancer (see Resources).

Menstrual cycle

The menstrual cycle (also referred to as the fertility cycle) is the process during which a follicle grows and develops, releasing a mature egg from one of the ovaries; meanwhile the endometrium prepares for a possible pregnancy. If a woman does not become pregnant, the endometrium is shed as a period (also known as menstruation). Periods are the result of the end of the cycle and mark the beginning of the next cycle. The menstrual cycle is controlled by the pituitary gland found at the base of the brain, which in turn controls the sex hormones – follicle-stimulating hormone (FSH), luteinizing hormone (LH), estrogen and progesterone. These chemical messengers are responsible for different actions during the cycle such as follicle development, ovulation, cycle length and periods (see Figure 2.4).

The first period a girl experiences is known as the menarche – the average age is around 11–13 years, but it can be earlier or later. Most girls will have started their periods by the age of 16. Early menstrual cycles are often irregular – meaning periods may be erratic in length, sometimes with very light bleeding, sometimes heavier bleeding. Over a few months, cycles generally start to settle down into a pattern as ovulation establishes itself. The length of the cycle and bleeding patterns will vary from woman to woman. Periods are often accompanied by low abdominal pain and cramps which can spread into the back or thighs. Cramps are due to contractions in the muscular uterine wall as it sheds the endometrium. Some periods may be more painful than others and this is normal, but if your periods are debilitating, talk to your doctor.

The number of days in the menstrual cycle – that is, how long it is – is calculated from the first day of the period to the day *before* the start of the next period. The average length of the menstrual cycle is around 28 days, plus or minus a few days. Many women have longer or shorter cycles, and this is normal. Few women have an absolutely regular menstrual cycle, and a variation of up to seven days is also very usual. It is important to remember that, although most women have menstrual cycles and the components are the same, how we each experience them can be very different. Many things can affect the cycle – factors such as age, diet, weight, stress, extreme exercise, illness and medication can cause the cycles to become irregular; sometimes periods may stop completely.

During each menstrual cycle, a woman is fertile (capable of becoming pregnant) for only a short time. Understanding this, and knowing how your menstrual cycle works, is the basis of fertility awareness.

The menstrual cycle can be divided into two main phases: the time *before* ovulation (pre-ovulatory phase), also known as the follicular phase; and the time *after* ovulation (post-ovulatory phase), also known as the luteal phase. However, for practical purposes, to identify the fertile and infertile times of the cycle, it is more appropriate to divide the menstrual cycle into **three phases:**

- **Early relatively infertile time**: The first phase lasts from the *start* of the period until the time when the follicles start growing – this phase is variable in length (from a few days up to several weeks). It is only considered *relatively* infertile.
- **Fertile time**: The second phase lasts from the time when the follicles start growing until about 48 hours after ovulation. The egg only survives for 24 hours, but if a second egg is released, this increases potential egg survival to 48 hours. Because sperm can survive for a number of days in a woman's body waiting for the egg to be released, there will be more days when sex can lead to pregnancy. The fertile time usually totals about ten days (including safety margins).
- **Late infertile time**: The third phase of the cycle extends from about three days after ovulation until the start of the next period. This phase is more constant in length and the safest time to have unprotected intercourse if pregnancy is to be avoided.

Figure 2.3 shows a representation of an average-length menstrual cycle with dark grey shading representing the period, light grey indicating the infertile times and white the fertile time. The fertile time starts as soon as there is any chance that sperm could survive in a woman's body – so, as soon as there are any cervical secretions. The fertile time ends 48 hours after ovulation – identified by a specific pattern in the temperature and cervical secretions. Note the arrows showing the variable length of time before ovulation compared with the constant length after ovulation.

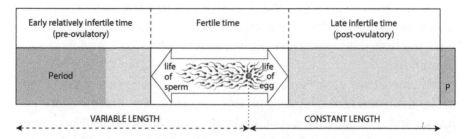

Figure 2.3 Menstrual cycle showing the fertile and infertile times
© Pyper & Knight, FertilityUK 2016

Step-by-step guide to the menstrual cycle

- The first day of the period is counted as day 1 of the cycle. Many women are confused about this and count the first day of the cycle if they get some blood spotting. Day 1 of the cycle is the first day of fresh red bleeding.
- During the first phase of the menstrual cycle, the pituitary gland produces FSH; this stimulates the development of follicles (which contain an egg) in the ovaries. Follicles produce the hormone oestradiol/estradiol (which is an estrogen); this causes the endometrium to start to thicken in preparation for a fertilized egg. Estrogen also affects the cervix, which becomes softer, its position becomes higher in the vagina and the cervical os opens slightly. The cervical secretions become thinner, wetter, clearer and stretchy. All these changes are designed to aid fertility and help sperm swim more easily through the cervix to reach an egg.
- Regardless of how long or short a woman's menstrual cycle is, ovulation (egg release from the ovary) will usually happen 10–16 days *before* the start of her next period. However, the time from the first day of the period to ovulation can vary considerably between women and between cycles. This is why women have different cycle lengths, some short, some long. A number of follicles containing eggs develop, but one follicle will mature and grow faster than the others. At this point, as estrogen levels rise and peak, FSH levels fall to prevent more follicles maturing and this triggers the production of luteinizing hormone (LH) which results in ovulation.
- Usually only one egg is released from one of the ovaries at ovulation. Occasionally, more than one egg is released, but if this happens, it will happen within 24 hours of the first egg being released. If more than one egg is released and is fertilized, it can lead to multiple pregnancy, such as non-identical twins. If one egg divides into two during embryo development, this can result in identical twins.

[1] The menstrual cycle is controlled by hormones. Follicle-stimulating hormone (FSH) causes the development of the egg follicles, which in turn produce the hormone estrogen. As the estrogen levels rise, this causes a surge in luteinizing hormone (LH) which ruptures the follicle and releases the egg at ovulation. The egg lives for up to 24 hours. After ovulation, the ovary produces progesterone. Estrogen and progesterone cause observable changes in the cervical secretions, the resting temperature and the cervix – the indicators of fertility.

[2] The period is the shedding of the endometrium. Approaching ovulation, the cervix produces secretions which nourish the sperm and help them to swim towards the egg. After ovulation, the secretions form a thick plug, blocking sperm penetration. The endometrium thickens in preparation for possible pregnancy.

[3] Estrogen and progesterone cause subtle changes in the cervix. It changes from low, firm, closed and tilted at the infertile time to high, soft, open and straight at the fertile time. After ovulation, the cervix changes back to low, firm, closed and tilted again. The cervical secretions change throughout the cycle. At first, they feel moist or sticky and look white or cloudy. Then they become wetter, transparent, slippery and stretchy (the most fertile time). After ovulation, the secretions change back to sticky then dry again.

[4] Sperm survival is around two to three days, but sperm can fertilize a woman's egg for longer and possibly up to seven days after intercourse when secretions are present. Allowing for the life of the egg, the fertile time usually lasts around ten days (including margins of safety). The days before the fertile time starts are only relatively infertile. The days after the fertile time ends are infertile – the safest time to have intercourse if you are avoiding pregnancy.

[5] The menstrual cycle is measured from the first day of one period to the day before the next period starts. The illustration shows a 28-day cycle. A woman's resting temperature rises slightly (app roximately 0.2 °C) after ovulation. It stays at the higher level until the start of the next period. A woman planning pregnancy has the highest chance of pregnancy from intercourse when the secretions are wet, transparent, slippery and stretchy. A woman who is avoiding pregnancy must consider that any secretions are potentially fertile.

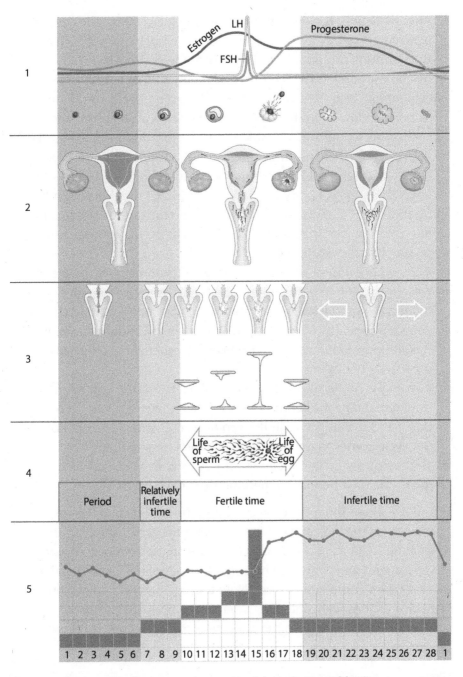

Figure 2.4 Menstrual cycle, hormonal control and the indicators of fertility
© Pyper & Knight, 2003 in collaboration with FertilityUK and IRH, Georgetown University

- After ovulation, the remains of the empty follicle form the corpus luteum, or 'yellow body' (because of its colour); this produces the hormone progesterone. This causes the endometrium to become spongy, thick and full of nutrients so that a fertilized egg can implant into it. At the same time, the cervix becomes firmer, its position lowers in the vagina and the cervical os closes. The cervical secretions become thick and sticky again forming a barrier to prevent further sperm getting through. At this time, the basal body temperature (BBT) or your resting temperature (which is a little lower than normal body temperature of 37 °C) rises very slightly by about 0.2 °C. This temperature marker illustrates that ovulation has occurred, not that ovulation is about to occur. This is the luteal phase or post-ovulation phase.
- If an egg is fertilized and implants into the endometrium, progesterone will remain high and no period will occur. The implanting embryo also triggers the production of the pregnancy hormone – human chorionic gonadotrophin (hCG), which helps maintain the endometrium. It is at this time that a woman may begin to experience some early pregnancy symptoms.
- If an egg is not fertilized, the body will reabsorb the egg naturally. Estrogen and progesterone levels will fall, the endometrium breaks down and is shed through the vagina as menstruation (a period) and this cycle comes to an end. The cycle then begins again.
- The menstrual cycle is a continuous cycle which occurs from menarche (first period) to menopause (final period).

Figure 2.4 shows the menstrual cycle and the influence of the sex hormones on the indicators of fertility. Note the arrow showing the fertile time – this starts as soon as there are any secretions to nourish the sperm and ends once the resting temperature has been sustained for three days at the higher level. Note that the time before ovulation is marked as 'relatively' infertile, whereas the time after ovulation is marked 'infertile' – this is the safest time for intercourse to avoid pregnancy.

Variations in cycle length

Figure 2.5 shows the variation in cycle length, illustrated by cycles of 22, 29 and 36 days. The time from ovulation to the *next* period remains

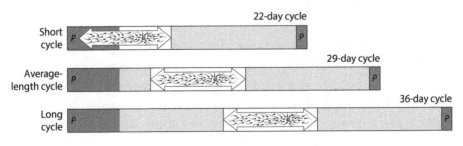

Figure 2.5 Variations in cycle length
© Pyper & Knight, FertilityUK 2016

constant at between ten and 16 days (average 14 days). Cycle lengths differ because of the variable length of the pre-ovulatory phase. Note the position of the fertile time arrow:

- In a short cycle of 22 days, ovulation occurs around day 8. Fertile secretions could be present during a period, and intercourse at that time could result in pregnancy. There are no early relatively infertile days.
- In an average-length cycle of 29 days, ovulation occurs around day 15 and there are a few early relatively infertile days.
- In a long cycle of 36 days, ovulation occurs around day 22 and the fertile time is delayed potentially giving many early relatively infertile days.

Fast facts

- Some menstrual cycles can be as short as 21 days, and some will be as long as 40 days or more.
- The average amount of menstrual blood lost during a period is 3–5 tablespoons – even if it might seem much more!
- A period usually lasts between three and eight days.
- Some women have pain around ovulation – known as *mittelschmerz* (German for 'middle pain').
- Bleeding or spotting between periods is not normal and should always be checked for infection or a gynaecology problem.

Menopause

When a woman is around 50 years old, her ovaries stop producing eggs. For some women, this occurs earlier, and for some later. Many women continue to have periods (sometimes quite regular periods) after they have stopped ovulating, so periods do not always indicate fertility. Menopause literally means the end of menstruation (the final period).

The time leading up to the menopause is called the perimenopause, and it is during this time that the hormonal and biological changes associated with the menopause begin. For example, periods can become heavier or lighter, more or less frequent, longer or shorter or stop altogether. Women may experience other symptoms such as hot flushes, vaginal dryness and changes in mood or libido. Although fertility during this time is extremely low, if you are still ovulating, it is possible to become pregnant. For this reason, women who do not want to become pregnant are advised to use contraception until they have not had a period or any bleeding for two years if under 50, and one year if over 50.

Men's bodies

Men's reproductive organs (Figure 2.6) are found entirely outside the body.

Penis

The penis is the external male reproductive organ. The penis has two main parts, the head (glans) and the shaft. A sleeve of skin called the foreskin surrounds and protects the delicate tip of the penis. Some men have this foreskin removed by surgery; this is called circumcision. The long hollow tube which runs from the bladder to the urinary opening is the urethra. Urine and semen come out of the urethra, but a complex valve system ensures that the function of urination and ejaculation of sperm cannot take place at the same time. Usually, the penis is soft and hangs down over the scrotum when not erect. When a man is sexually excited (and at other times too) the erectile tissue fills with blood and the penis becomes stiff, grows longer and wider and sticks outwards

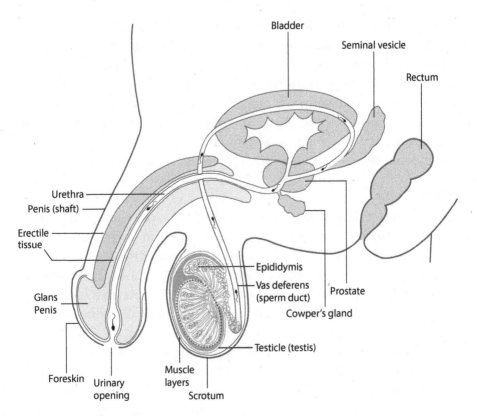

Figure 2.6 Male reproductive organs (genitals)

and upwards from his body. The foreskin, when present, slides back to leave the head of the penis completely exposed.

The shape of an erect penis varies, although it usually curves upwards slightly, and may point slightly to one side. Penis size also varies, but not by very much. Adult penis size is usually between 8.5 cm and 10.5 cm (3–4 inches) long when soft, and between 15 and 18 cm (6–7 inches) when hard.

Testicles and scrotum

The testicles are the male equivalent of a woman's ovaries. Men have two testicles (testes), about the size of two small plums. They are contained and protected in a soft pouch of skin called the scrotum. The scrotum hangs outside the body just behind the penis and between the legs. Inside the testicles, sperm are made and the male hormone – testosterone – is produced.

Sperm are very sensitive to heat – the average body temperature (37 °C) is too hot to produce healthy sperm. If the testes get too hot, the scrotum muscle relaxes and it drops down to cool off. When too cold, the scrotum shrinks closer to the body to keep warm. If the temperature is too hot or too cold, sperm cell production can be adversely affected.

Testosterone is responsible for sperm production. It is also important for male growth and sex drive and controls male characteristics such as hair growth, deepening of the voice, body shape and muscle build.

Sperm

Inside each testicle are many tightly coiled tubes. Sperm are produced here in a continuous process. The sperm travel along the tiny tubes to a larger coiled tube called the epididymis, which is at the top of the testicle. They stay here while they gain their motility (ability to move) and they are fully mature and ready to be ejaculated. Sperm are microscopic and are made up of a head, middle and a tail – they look rather like tadpoles. Sperm are the smallest cell in the human body. The head carries the chromosomes (genes that determine what we look like – see Chapter 8) The middle section contains the energy to nourish the sperm and the tail enables the sperm to move. Sperm are produced every day in a continuous process from puberty to the end of a man's life.

Fast facts

- Men produce many millions of sperm every day, so they do not run out.
- It takes about 70 days for a sperm to develop and a little longer to mature, but as the production of sperm is a continuous process there are always plenty of sperm at any one time.
- Sperm are excellent swimmers. In the right conditions, some sperm will enter the cervix within minutes of intercourse and move through to the uterus in two to seven hours.
- The average ejaculation contains 2–4 ml of semen (about a teaspoon) and each millilitre contains around 100 million sperm.
- The average sperm survival is around two to three days, but sometimes sperm can live for up to seven days in really good conditions.

Ejaculation

At ejaculation sperm are propelled through the vas deferens (sperm ducts) to the penis and out of the body through the urethra. On the way, fluid from the seminal vesicles and prostate gland is added to the sperm. This helps nourish and transport them and gives seminal fluid (semen) its creamy white appearance.

To prepare for ejaculation a small amount of lubricating fluid known as pre-ejaculatory fluid is produced from Cowper's glands. This fluid leaks out of the penis before ejaculation and may contain sperm. When a man ejaculates, the muscles of the penis contract forcing the semen out of the penis in spurts. Straight after ejaculation the fluid is thick but it becomes liquid very quickly, which helps release the sperm. Although many sperm are released, only about 100 sperm survive the journey in the woman's reproductive system and only one will finally penetrate the ovum (egg) to achieve fertilization and pregnancy.

Understanding conception – getting pregnant

Studies that accurately measure hormone levels in the urine show that there are only six days in the menstrual cycle when intercourse could result in pregnancy – that is from five days before ovulation to the day of ovulation itself. In Figure 2.7 you can see that there are no pregnancies six days before or one day after ovulation. The highest chance of pregnancy is on the day of ovulation and the two days before – with around 30 per cent chance at that time. It is not possible to detect ovulation so precisely with home test kits or by observing fertility indicators. The aim is to find the start and end of the fertile time – this usually totals around ten days which allows for margins of error.

For a woman to become pregnant (conceive), an egg must be fertilized by a sperm and become implanted in the endometrium (lining of the uterus). Conception is a process that begins with fertilization and ends with successful implantation of a fertilized egg in the uterus so pregnancy can begin (Figure 2.8).

Usually, but not always, egg and sperm meet through sexual intercourse between a man and a woman (natural conception). If penetrative sex is not possible, the egg may be fertilized artificially by a sperm using some form of assisted conception. The simplest form of

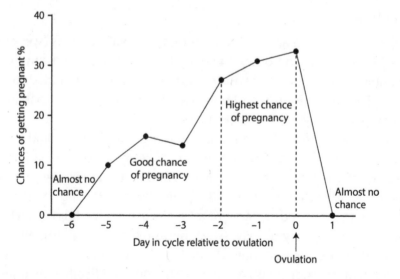

Figure 2.7 Chances of conception in relation to the day of ovulation

(Adapted from Wilcox, A.J., et al., 1995, Timing of sexual intercourse in relation to ovulation. *New England Journal of Medicine* 333(23): 1517–21)

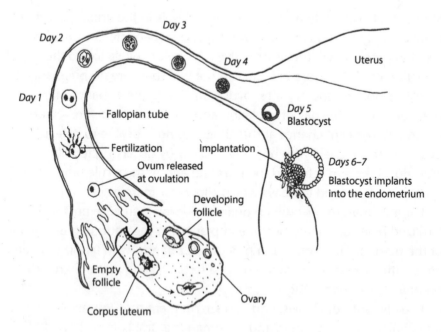

Figure 2.8 Conception: from fertilization to implantation

assistance is through self-insemination (home-insemination). This can be used by single women, women in same-sex relationships, where a man or woman has a disability creating difficulties with intercourse, or where intercourse cannot be completed for physical or psychological reasons. There are many different types of assisted conception – IUI (intra-uterine insemination) and IVF (in-vitro fertilization) being the most commonly known. For more information on assisted conception, see Chapter 9 and Resources.

Steps to conception

- The ovary releases an egg, which is picked up by one of the two fallopian tubes. The tiny hairs (cilia) in the tube and their wave-like contractions help the egg travel along the fallopian tube where it may meet a sperm within minutes or hours of ovulation. An egg only lives for up to 24 hours (potential of 48 hours, total egg survival time if there is a second ovulation), so the chances of fertilization are increased if sperm are ready and waiting. This means having regular sexual intercourse two to three times a week helps to ensure there are always available sperm.
- Only one sperm will be able to penetrate the egg. Sperm produce a special substance that dissolves the outer covering of the egg. Once the sperm has entered the egg, the egg undergoes a chemical change, which prevents any other sperm getting in. The chromosomes from the sperm and the egg fuse together. This is fertilization.
- Inside the fertilized egg, the cells start to divide and continue to divide as the fertilized egg travels down the fallopian tube into the uterus. By three days it is a ball of cells rather like a very tiny blackberry, and by five days (the blastocyst stage) it has about 100 cells (see Figure 2.8).
- Once in the uterus, the blastocyst (very early embryo) starts to settle in and uses a special glue-like mechanism to attach itself to the thick, nutritious endometrium. It then starts to penetrate through the surface of the endometrium to connect with the mother's blood supply. Successful implantation has now taken place, conception is complete and pregnancy begins.

- Many eggs, even when fertilized successfully, do not implant – this is normal. If this happens, the fertilized egg is shed when the woman has a period. It requires at least ten days following ovulation to complete the implantation process. If a fertilized egg gets stuck in the fallopian tube (perhaps because of a blockage) and tries to implant, this may result in an ectopic pregnancy.

Fast facts

- Conception is a process that starts with fertilization and ends with implantation.
- The egg can be fertilized by sperm that have been ejaculated up to seven days before.
- The egg has special places on its outside covering that attract sperm.
- It takes about 15 minutes for the sperm to cross the outer membrane and enter the egg.
- It takes a couple an average of three to six months to conceive, if they are having intercourse frequently (two to three times a week) during their fertile time.
- Women over 30 years old may take longer to conceive.

Sex and conception

For most couples, sexual activity including intercourse is usually a pleasurable and emotionally bonding experience and is not purely about reproduction. Many couples will spend years having sex for pleasure using contraception to avoid pregnancy. When the focus of sex switches to having a baby, it is a time to enjoy having sex without having to think about the need for contraception. It is important to maintain that pleasure and to try not to lose the spontaneity because you now want to become pregnant.

For natural conception to occur, a man needs to be able to get an erection and insert his erect penis into the woman's vagina and ejaculate inside her. The whole mechanism of sexual response is a reflex activity, which works most successfully in a state of relaxation.

Sexual response in men and women

Sexual response can be divided into four phases: excitement or arousal, plateau, orgasm and resolution. These phases are essentially the same for men and women but with subtle differences between the sexes.

- **Sexual arousal:** Sexual stimulation activates sensitive nerve endings causing an increase in blood flow to the pelvic area. For men, the spongy tissue of the penis fills with blood and the penis becomes erect. For women, the clitoris increases in size and the smooth inner vaginal lips become fuller and are moistened with a clear lubricating fluid.
- **Plateau phase:** With continued stimulation, the penis becomes firmer, the testicles are drawn closer to the body and a drop of clear lubricating pre-ejaculatory fluid may be noticed at the tip of the penis. For a woman, as sexual arousal and tension increases, the inner vaginal lips become softer and more engorged, the clitoris swells further in size, the vagina becomes more lubricated, the cervix is pulled up further and the top part of the vagina 'balloons' to form a shape which will hold the sperm in contact with the cervix.
- **Orgasm:** With further stimulation, the man's seminal vesicles and prostate gland contract adding fluid for the sperm, the urethra contracts rhythmically and the seminal fluid is then ejaculated. Nearly all men experience an orgasm at the same time as ejaculation, although its intensity may vary. Orgasm is felt as an intense, pleasurable sensation of a sudden build-up and release of sexual tension. A woman may or may not reach orgasm during intercourse; this is often dependent on good sexual technique and direct clitoral stimulation. Female orgasm is similar to the man's – a woman will experience a build-up and release of sexual tension lasting up to about 15 seconds and she may feel her vagina contracting rhythmically. She may also feel pleasurable contractions of her uterus. Men and women experience a surge of the hormone oxytocin at orgasm, which induces a sense of total relaxation and calm – it is often known as the love or bonding hormone.

! Myths about female orgasm

The key difference between male and female orgasm is that a woman is physically able to go on to experience further orgasm(s) within a matter of seconds. The pattern of sexual response will vary from one woman to another and within the same woman from one sexual experience to another. A woman may have a short plateau phase followed by a single orgasm; a longer plateau phase and multiple orgasms; or a plateau phase with no orgasm and a much slower resolution phase. Although men may find it hard to relate to this, all of these experiences can be deeply satisfying for a woman.

Orgasm is not necessary for a woman to get pregnant; however, research clearly shows that the uterine contractions associated with orgasm help to suck up the semen making conception more likely. It is well recognized that only about half of all women experience an orgasm from vaginal penetration alone, so time for more creative lovemaking can be time well spent. Some women rarely or never achieve orgasm (anorgasmia) but may still enjoy a fulfilling sex life. If you are concerned about any aspect of your sex life, see your GP or find a psychosexual therapist, through the College of Sexual and Relationship Therapists (COSRT) – see Resources.

- **Resolution phase:** As the intense pleasure of orgasm is past, there is usually a sense of calm and sexual fulfilment. In men, the blood flow that increased the congestion in the pelvic organs drains away and the erection is lost, the testicles descend and the scrotum becomes softer and looser. Similarly, during this phase, the woman's pelvic organs return to their pre-aroused state.

The time taken before a man can become sexually aroused again will vary from a few minutes to hours for a young man to a longer interval as a man gets older – this is known as the refractory period (recovery phase). Women do not have a refractory period in the same way and, if stimulated appropriately, may go on to have further orgasms quite quickly.

3

Finding your fertile time

Fertility awareness is empowering. Whether you learn purely for interest, to plan or avoid pregnancy, it gives you a better understanding of your menstrual cycles and puts you in control of your fertility. To find the fertile time in your cycle, you will need to take a few moments each day to observe your indicators (signs and symptoms) of fertility.

Most women today have smartphones and use a variety of apps for many aspects of their lives. If you have been using a period tracker or any kind of fertility app, you can continue to use your app, but it is preferable to record your observations on a fertility chart (see the blank charts at the end of the book). Over time, you should start to see a pattern emerging which will give you confidence in your ability to understand your fertility. You can see how your new understanding of the fertile time compares with the predictions made by your app.

Indicators of fertility

There are four major indicators of fertility:

1 Cycle length
2 Cervical secretions
3 Resting temperature
4 Cervical changes.

This chapter looks at each indicator in turn and considers its role in planning and avoiding pregnancy.

1 Cycle length

Cycle length is calculated from the first day of one period to the day before the next period starts. Keep an ongoing record of your cycle lengths. Provided your cycles are fairly regular, you can get a *rough* estimate of your fertile time by using a calculation based on the length of your last 12 cycles – the *S minus 20* and *L minus 10* rules.

S minus 20 and L minus 10 rules

From your last 12 cycle lengths, work out your shortest cycle (S) and longest cycle (L). Then subtract 20 from the shortest cycle and 10 from the longest to find your first and last fertile day.

S minus 20 = first fertile day
L minus 10 = last fertile day

For example: If your last 12 cycles were 29, 26, 27, 31, 29, 28, 26, 29, 30, 31, 28 and 27 days, the shortest cycle is 26 days and the longest is 31 days. 26 – 20 = 6 and 31 – 10 = 21.

Your fertile time is therefore potentially from days 6 to 21 inclusive.

Update your calculation at the end of each cycle so you use your 12 most recent cycles.

The fertile time based on past cycle lengths is quite wide. In the example, if you were going to have a short cycle you could possibly conceive from having sex as early as day 6, but if you were going to have a long cycle, you could conceive from sex as late as day 21.

Using cycle length calculation alone

- **To conceive**: The calculation gives a *rough* idea of the fertile time which helps make sure you are covering all bases, but the secretions will help you to target intercourse more precisely (see below).
- **To avoid pregnancy**: The S minus 20 rule gives an early warning of the *start* of the fertile time (see below), but the L minus 10 rule is not sufficiently accurate for avoiding pregnancy; you need to cross-check temperature with secretions to find the *end* of your fertile time (see below).

2 Cervical secretions

Cervical secretions are key to fertility awareness whether planning or avoiding pregnancy – they also give more general information about reproductive and sexual health. Normal healthy secretions are white, creamy-coloured, cloudy or transparent – they have no smell. By comparison, abnormal vaginal discharges are discoloured and they may have an offensive smell – you might also notice redness, soreness or itching around the vulva. If you observe any change from your normal pattern of secretions, see your doctor or go to your local sexual health clinic (see the paragraph on sexual health checks in Chapter 8).

How secretions encourage or block sperm

It helps to understand a little about the structure of the cervix and its secretions and the effect of the hormones estrogen and progesterone. The cervical canal, which is 2–3 cm long, produces secretions along its length but their characteristics change during the cycle. High-resolution images show that when sperm enter the cervical canal, they are confronted by a complex 3D maze of interwoven mucus strands – the width of these strands and the size of the gaps between them varies controlling whether or not sperm can pass.

- At the fertile time (when estrogen levels are high), the mucus strands are thin and the gaps between them are wide, allowing sperm to swim through easily (see Figure 3.1 – magnified image on left). The wide gaps between the strands form swimming channels which guide sperm through the cervical canal. Sperm can survive for up to seven days in these alkaline conditions waiting for the egg to be released.
- At the infertile times of the cycle, the mucus strands are thicker and the gaps between them are too small for sperm to push their way through – sperm are left to perish in the acidic vagina. The mucus strands are at their thickest and most densely packed after ovulation when progesterone levels are at their highest (see Figure 3.1 – magnified image on right).

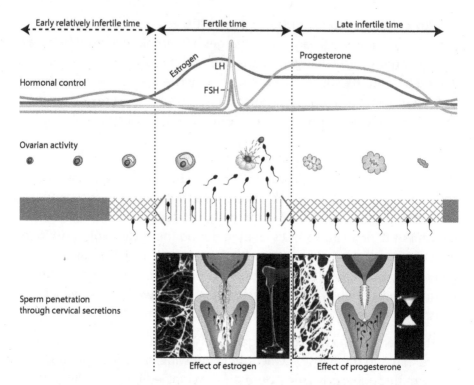

Figure 3.1 Hormonal effect on secretions and sperm penetration at the fertile time
© Pyper & Knight, FertilityUK 2016

Changes in cervical secretions through the cycle

The changes in secretions follow a recognizable pattern through the menstrual cycle, but this varies slightly from woman to woman and from one cycle to the next.

Early (pre-ovulatory) relatively infertile time

After your period, you may notice a few dry days – you feel dry at the vulva with no visible secretions. If you have a long cycle, you may have many dry days; but if you have a short cycle, you may not have *any* dry days.

Fertile time

As the egg follicles grow and the estrogen levels rise, you may become aware of a feeling of moistness or stickiness at the vulva and see small amounts of white or creamy-coloured secretions. If you gently test the secretions with your fingertip, they hold their shape and break easily. The secretions increase in amount, become thinner, cloudy and slightly stretchy – you may feel wetter at the vulva. As estrogen levels continue to rise (with approaching ovulation), you may be aware of a feeling of slipperiness or lubrication at the vulva. You may notice lots of thin, watery, transparent (clear) secretions, rather like raw egg white. These highly fertile secretions may stretch for several centimetres before they break (see Figure 3.1)

One of the most significant days is **peak day** – it is called 'peak' because, rather like a mountain peak, it is the high point of your cycle (close to ovulation). Peak day is the LAST day that you either feel or see the wetter, slippery, transparent, stretchy secretions. You can only know which day was peak in retrospect, because on the day after peak there is a distinct change back to stickiness or dryness again. Peak day is not necessarily the day with the most profuse wet secretions – this frequently occurs one or two days before the peak. Peak day is always the LAST day when secretions show the most fertile characteristics. You remain fertile for three full days after peak.

Late (post-ovulatory) infertile time

The day after peak, you will notice that the wet/slippery feeling has gone and the vulva feels sticky or dry again – this change happens quite quickly from one day to the next (due to progesterone following ovulation). You will then be aware of a feeling of dryness or slight stickiness until your next period starts. The late infertile time starts on the fourth day after peak.

There are three key steps to monitoring your secretions:

- Observing
- Recording
- Interpreting.

Observing secretions

Observe your secretions at intervals throughout the day – the easiest way is each time you go to the toilet. You recognize secretions by sensation (feeling) at the vulva, appearance (the look) describing the colour, and by the finger-test (touch) describing the consistency/texture (see Figure 3.2)

- **Sensation**: Sensation is important but it is often the most difficult to learn. Think for a moment about how you sense that your period has started – it is hard to describe it but you 'just know'. In exactly the same way, you can learn to recognize the sensation that tells you whether or not there are any secretions at the vulva. You might describe this as a distinct feeling of dryness or 'nothingness', or a feeling of dampness/moistness, stickiness, wetness, slipperiness or lubrication.
- **Appearance**: Use soft white toilet paper to blot or wipe your vulva. You may just see dampness on the paper from vaginal moistness or urine. Urine soaks into the paper while any cervical secretions appear raised as a blob. Note the colour: white, creamy, cloudy or transparent. If you see secretions in your pants, they will have dried slightly causing some alteration in characteristics and colour.
- **Finger test**: Lightly apply your fingertip to the secretion on the toilet paper, then gently pull it away to test its capacity to stretch. It may feel sticky and break easily, or smoother and slippery like raw egg white and stretch between your finger and thumb for up to several centimetres before it breaks. This stretchiness, known as the spinn-barkeit effect, shows that the secretions are highly fertile.

First cycle of charting

It is helpful to avoid intercourse completely on your first cycle of charting to give you time to recognize your own pattern of secretions without confusion from seminal fluid. Once you gain some experience, you will be able to distinguish between different fluids. If you have intercourse in the evening, you may still feel some wetness from residual seminal fluid the following morning, but by midday this will be gone and you have the rest of the day to observe your secretions. Intercourse in the morning/daytime can make it more difficult to observe secretions, which is why there may be times when it is safest to restrict intercourse to the evenings.

Recording secretions on the chart

If you are trying to conceive, the planning pregnancy chart has space to record four cycles (see Appendix). If you are avoiding pregnancy, record your secretions on a combined indicator chart (see Appendix).

Sensation at vulva	Finger-test	Appearance
Moist or sticky	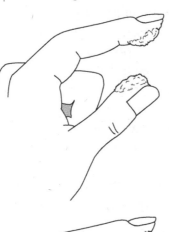	**Early secretion** Scant, white, sticky, holds its shape
Wetter		Increasing amounts, thinner, cloudy, slightly stretchy
Slippery	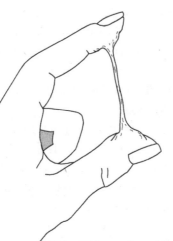	**Highly fertile secretion** Profuse, thin transparent, stretchy (like raw egg white)

Note: All types of secretion are potentially fertile.

Figure 3.2 Characteristics of cervical secretions

1 Record your observations on the chart in the evening. Consider sensation, appearance and finger-test.
2 Shade in the appropriate box:
   a Period, including blood spotting
   b Dry – no secretions seen or felt
   c Moist, white, cloudy, sticky
   d Wet, slippery, transparent, stretchy.
3 Mark peak day – the last day in the top box (box 4) – by extending the shading upwards to form a 'chimney' effect. You will only know which day is peak when you notice a distinct change the following day as the secretions become thicker and stickier again or you feel dry. Notice that the day after peak is recorded in a lower box (either box 3 or 2).
4 Each time you have intercourse, circle the appropriate day of the cycle. Note if you use a barrier method (e.g. C for condoms).

Interpreting changes in secretions

Figure 3.3 shows a typical pattern of secretions. The boxes are numbered for explanatory purposes from box 1 (bottom box) to box 4 (top). In this example, the period (box 1) lasts five days, then days 6 and 7 are dry (box 2). Day 8 shows the first sign of moist, white, cloudy, sticky secretions (first day in box 3) – the fertile time has started (note the heavier line between boxes 2 and 3). On days 9 and 10, the secretions still fit the description in box 3, but on day 11 they are wet, slippery, transparent and stretchy (box 4). Day 13 is peak day (last day in box 4). Peak could only be confirmed on day 14 when the secretions were sticky again (box 3). From day 15 until the start of the next period was dry. Note the 'count of 3' after peak. Writing '1, 2, 3' in the top box on the three days following peak ensures that there are no further secretions which would fit the description in box 4. The fertile time starts on day 8 (first sign of any secretions) and lasts until day 16 (three full days after peak). Note the fertile time arrow from day 8 to 16 inclusive.

Only shade in *one* box to describe your secretions at the end of each day. When considering which box, shade the box which best describes the *most fertile* characteristics you have seen over the course of the day. For example: if you noticed sticky white secretions in the morning but, by evening, they felt wetter and slightly stretchy, shade in the top box.

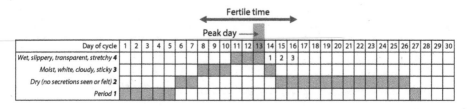

Figure 3.3 Typical pattern of secretions through the menstrual cycle

The change back after peak day is important – the secretions on the day following peak should not show *any* characteristics which would fit into the top box.

Using cervical secretions alone

- **To conceive**: the secretions give all the information you need about your fertile time.
  - The fertile time starts at the first sign of any secretions.
  - Intercourse on days of wetter, transparent, slippery, stretchy secretions carries the highest chance of pregnancy.
  - The fertile time ends three days after peak (see above).
- **To avoid pregnancy**: FAMs are more effective using a combination of indicators. Cross-check the first sign of secretions with a calculation to find the start of your fertile time and cross-check the secretions with temperature to find the end of your fertile time (see below).

3 Resting temperature

Resting temperature (sometimes referred to as waking temperature) is body temperature at rest after a night's sleep. Changes in resting temperature help to *confirm* ovulation. After ovulation, progesterone from the corpus luteum causes a slight rise in temperature. The rise helps to identify the *end* of your fertile time. Temperature has no value in predicting ovulation.

In a cycle where ovulation occurs, the temperature has two distinct levels: in the early part of the cycle, it will be at the lower level; then,

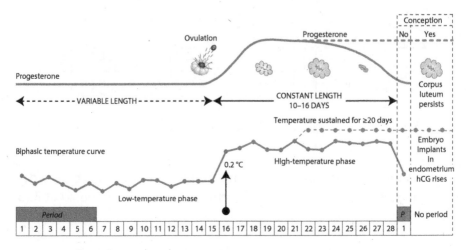

Figure 3.4 Effect of progesterone on resting temperature

after ovulation, it rises by around 0.2 degrees Celsius (0.2 °C) to the higher level where it remains until the next period starts.

- If conception occurs, the corpus luteum continues to produce progesterone, the endometrium is maintained (to support a pregnancy) and the temperature stays at the higher level.
- If there is no conception, the corpus luteum degenerates, the progesterone level falls and the temperature drops back to the lower level around the start of the next period (see Figure 3.4).

To monitor your temperature, you need a thermometer, chart, a ruler, black and red pens.

Thermometers

Use a battery-operated Celsius digital thermometer and follow the manufacturer's instructions. Make sure the thermometer has:

- an intermittent bleep while the thermometer is registering
- a continuous bleep when the temperature has stabilized (usually less than one minute)
- a last memory recall (so you don't have to write your temperature down immediately)
- a low-battery warning light.

Digital thermometers are virtually unbreakable. They have an easy-to-read electronic display. Some record to two decimal places and others to one. One decimal place (e.g., 36.7) is sufficient and preferable (additional information is confusing and unnecessary). A good digital thermometer should cost around £10 – you do not need an expensive computerized thermometer. Ear and forehead thermometers and axillary (underarm) temperatures are not reliable enough for fertility purposes.

Celsius vs Fahrenheit

Digital thermometers are widely available through pharmacies and online – most are in degrees Celsius, although in the USA, Fahrenheit may be more readily available. Some thermometers include both scales. As this book is written from the perspective of a Celsius scale, it is much simpler if you find a Celsius thermometer. If you do wish to use Fahrenheit, remember that 0.1 degrees Celsius is roughly equivalent to 0.2 degrees Fahrenheit. So, when the text refers to the third high temperature being at least 0.2 degrees Celsius higher, this will be 0.4 degrees Fahrenheit higher. Consistency is vital – choose your thermometer and if ever you want to switch from one temperature scale to the other, never switch during the same cycle, make the change at the start of a new cycle.

Charts

The blank chart (see Appendix) can be copied for personal use. This easy-to-use chart includes space for recording your name, age, chart number, dates and days of the week, current and past cycle lengths, temperature route and target time, a Celsius temperature grid (with Celsius in bold text and Fahrenheit in italics) and boxes to record secretions and cervix. Use the comments box to note disturbances. Blank charts and instructions can also be downloaded free from the FertilityUK site at www.fertilityuk.org. Figure 3.5 shows a completed chart with a digital thermometer.

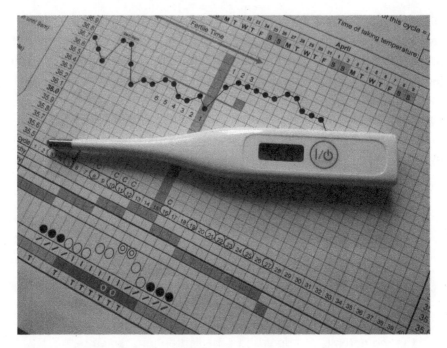

Figure 3.5 Completed chart with a digital thermometer

Recording the period and cycle length

The chart spans 40 days with cycle days numbered 1–40 across the bottom.

- Indicate the days of your period by shading the appropriate box.
- Day 1 is the first day of the period (fresh red bleed).
  - If you start a red bleed at any time during the day (before bedtime) count that day as day 1 and transfer that morning's temperature to a new chart.
  - If you start a red bleed overnight and notice the next morning, then that morning is counted as day 1.
- Consider any light bleeding or spotting before a red bleed starts as the end of the previous cycle. Use dots instead of solid shading.
- Measure your cycle length from the first day of one period up until the day *before* the next period starts. You will only know the length of the cycle once your *next* period starts.
- Record your cycle length in the box at the top right of the chart.
- Keep a record of cycle lengths to estimate your shortest cycle over the past 12 cycles (see above).

Recording and charting resting temperature

- Take your temperature at about the same time every morning – immediately as you wake up, before you get out of bed or do anything. Choose your target time – normally the time you set your alarm on weekdays. If you have to get up during the night, aim to have at least three undisturbed hours resting back in bed before taking your temperature.
- Most women take their temperature by mouth (orally) but some prefer an internal temperature (vaginal or rectal). If you decide to change route, do so at the start of the cycle and note it on the chart. Internal temperatures will be slightly higher than oral.
  - **Oral temperatures**: Place the thermometer under the fleshy part of your tongue in contact with the floor of your mouth. Gently close your lips and breathe normally through your nose.
  - **Vaginal temperatures**: Insert the thermometer gently into your vagina for about 4–5 cm. Slide your finger alongside the thermometer to make sure it is correctly positioned.
  - **Rectal temperatures**: Smear the thermometer probe with a little lubricant. Lie on your side with your knees drawn up and gently insert the thermometer into the rectum for about 2–3 cm. Rectal temperatures are rarely used in the UK.
- Mark the reading on the chart by drawing a dot in the *centre* of the appropriate square. Join the dots to form a continuous graph. If you miss a day, just leave a gap – do *not* join non-consecutive dots. If you forget to take your temperature around the time of the rise, you may not have enough readings to interpret your chart.

If your thermometer records to two decimal places, always round *down* (only record the first decimal place) – for example, if the thermometer reads 36.87, record this as 36.8 °C. Your logical brain may want to average up to 36.9, but this could result in false high readings. The important thing is to be consistent.

Remember that temperatures can be disrupted by disturbances such as late nights, alcohol or oversleeping. Use a red pen to highlight disturbed readings and note any explanations in the comments box.

Setting your target time

You need to be consistent with the time you take your temperature. Body temperature works on a circadian (24-hour) rhythm: it is at its lowest at around 4 a.m., then it rises steadily by approximately 0.1 °C every hour that you stay in bed. Provided you take your temperature within an hour of your target time (30 minutes each side), this is still within range. For example: if you normally set your alarm for 7 a.m., anytime from 06:30 until 07:30 is within target.

If you take your temperature outside your target time, make the following adjustments:

- Later temperature: count *down* one square for each hour later that it has been taken. For example: if the alarm is normally set for 07:00 on weekdays, but you sleep in until 09:00 on Sunday morning, adjust the temperature *downwards* by two squares
- Earlier temperature: count *up* one square for each hour earlier. For example: if the alarm is normally set for 07:00, but you had an early start at 05:30, adjust the reading *upwards* by one square.

With experience, most women can manage time differences with confidence but you should only make such adjustments in collaboration with an accredited practitioner.

Common errors with temperature

Errors in taking or recording your temperature could result in abnormally high or low readings. Common errors include:

- Not leaving the thermometer in place for long enough
- Changing temperature-taking time with no explanation
- Changing temperature-taking route mid-cycle
- Changing thermometer mid-cycle – there may be a slight discrepancy between thermometers
- Battery failure
- Faulty thermometer.

If you have ruled out these errors and your readings do not improve, you may need to switch to a vaginal temperature.

Interpreting temperature readings
Biphasic charts

A cycle in which ovulation occurs (ovulatory cycle) is characterized by a biphasic chart (two levels): the temperature stays at the lower level until just after ovulation when it rises by about 0.2 °C. The rise usually occurs abruptly between one day and the next. The temperature remains at the higher level until just before or at the start of the next period.

If you want to avoid pregnancy, you can't resume intercourse immediately after the temperature rise – you need to allow sufficient time for egg survival. The egg can be fertilized for up to 24 hours after ovulation. As there is a possibility of a second ovulation (as with non-identical twins), allow another 24 hours giving **48 hours' total egg survival time**. To ensure that 48 hours has elapsed, wait for three temperatures at the higher level. This is the *3 over 6* rule.

The 3 over 6 rule

The 3 over 6 rule identifies the end of the fertile time (beginning of late infertile time): There must be three undisturbed high temperatures above the level of the previous six low temperatures.
   To apply the 3 over 6 rule:

- Draw a horizontal line (coverline) on the line immediately above the highest of the low-phase temperatures.
- Draw a vertical line to form a cross dividing the low- and high-phase temperatures.
- Number the high temperatures 1–3 and the low temperatures 1–6 (in reverse order). For emphasis, write 'high' numbers above and 'low' numbers below (see Figure 3.6).
- The three high temperatures must be undisturbed and they must all be above the level of the six low temperatures.
- The temperature rise need only be 0.1 °C, but the third high temperature must be a minimum of 0.2 °C above the low temperatures. A single hatched box drawn in the square just above the coverline ensures that the third high reading is at least 0.2 °C above the low temperatures.
- If the third high temperature is not at least 0.2 °C, wait for a fourth high temperature which just has to be above the coverline.

45

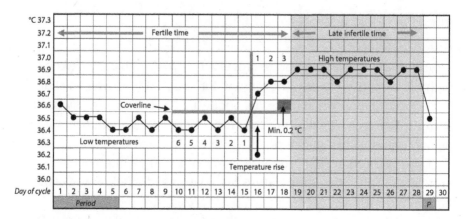

Figure 3.6 Biphasic chart showing the late infertile time

In Figure 3.6, note that the fertile time extends from day 1 until the third high temperature – temperature does not give any warning of the *start* of the fertile time. The fertile time *ends* after the third high temperature and the rest of the cycle will be infertile – the late infertile time. If you are avoiding pregnancy, double-check that all your high temperatures occur after peak day (see Figure 3.13 and the guidelines that follow).

Different types of temperature rise

The temperature rises in one of three ways:

- **Abrupt rise**: rises abruptly between one day and the next (most common)
- **Slow rise**: rises slowly over several days
- **Step rise**: rises by 0.1 °C or 0.2 °C then stays at that level for 48 hours before progressing another step.

Figure 3.7 shows the different types of temperature rise. There must be three temperatures in the upper right quadrant and at least six in the lower left (3 over 6 rule). Note the hatched box which ensures that the third high temperature is at least 0.2 °C. Figure 4.5 shows an example of waiting for the fourth high temperature when the third is not at least 0.2 °C.

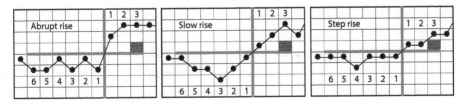

Figure 3.7 Types of temperature rise

Is there a dip before the rise?

It is common to see illustrations of charts showing a temperature dip (labelled 'ovulation') before the rise. In practice, few charts show a dip and there are many other reasons for dips (e.g. getting up earlier or taking painkillers). Forget about dips. It is the *rise* in temperature which is associated with ovulation.

Variations in the day of temperature rise

The overall length of cycles varies, but it is the time before ovulation which is most varied. As the temperature rise occurs 10–16 days before

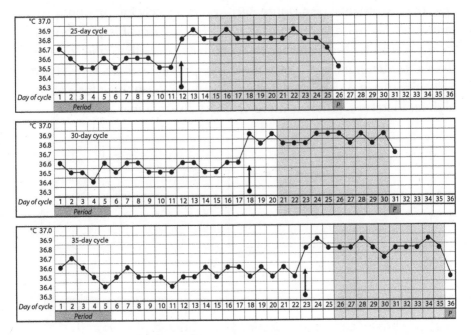

Figure 3.8 Variations in the day of the temperature rise

the start of the next period, it follows that the rise occurs earlier in shorter cycles and later in longer cycles. Figure 3.8 shows cycles of 25, 30 and 35 days. In the short cycle, the temperature rise (first high temperature) occurs on day 12 as shown by the upward arrow. In the average-length cycle, the rise occurs on day 18; and in the long cycle, it occurs on day 23. If you have a cycle of more than 40 days, join two charts together to see when (or if) the rise occurs. Figure 5.3 shows a long cycle after stopping the pill.

If you are avoiding pregnancy, always assume that there will be a temperature rise and wait for the rise – however delayed. In a cycle of 42 days, for example, the temperature may not rise until around day 30 (after the time you might have expected your period). In some cycles there may be no rise – see the monophasic charts section later in this chapter.

Temperature spike

A temperature spike is a *single* recording which is 0.2 °C or more above the one on each side (its immediate neighbours). You may notice a spike if you drink alcohol or have a lie-in. Sometimes there may be no apparent reason. Circle the spike using a red pen so that you can easily spot the disturbance (see Figure 3.9). You can safely ignore one spike in the six low-phase temperatures, but wherever possible you should have a reason for the disturbance. If you have more than one spike in the six low temperatures, you cannot interpret your chart. If you have a disturbance in one of your three high temperatures, wait for a fourth high temperature. (There is more on chart disturbances below.)

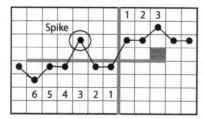 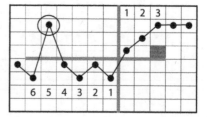

Figure 3.9 Temperature spike

Conception cycles

In a cycle where conception occurs, the temperature stays at the higher level and there is no period. Some women notice a second rise

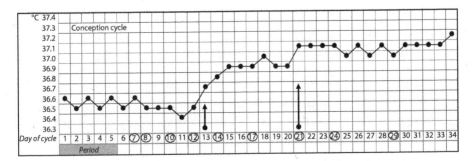

Figure 3.10 Conception cycle showing a sustained high temperature

in temperature about a week after the ovulation rise – this is due to the increased progesterone following implantation. If the temperature stays at the higher level for 20 days or more, conception is most likely. Figure 3.10 shows a conception cycle – note the second rise in temperature on day 21. The cycle is ongoing with more than 20 high temperatures – it's time to do a pregnancy test!

Short luteal phases

Cycles in which the luteal (post-ovulation) phase is less than ten days may have insufficient time for implantation. You can only work out the length of your luteal phase when you get your period, but if you have fewer than ten raised temperatures you have a short luteal phase. Short luteal phases occur sporadically in women of all ages but they are more common in adolescents, after childbirth and approaching the menopause. They are also common if you are stressed. Figure 3.11 shows a 21-day cycle: the temperature rise occurs on day 14 but the next period starts on day 22 – the luteal phase is only eight days, so it may be unable to sustain a pregnancy.

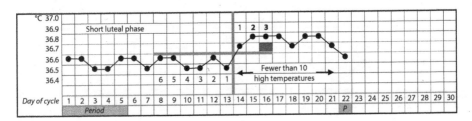

Figure 3.11 Short luteal phase

A short luteal phase can occur in a cycle of any length. For example, if the temperature rise occurs on day 27, but the next period starts on day 36, the overall cycle length is long, but the luteal phase is short.

- **To conceive**: If you have fewer than ten high temperatures for three or more consecutive cycles, talk to your doctor. The fertility chart provides helpful information which may indicate the need for further tests (such as a blood test to check your mid-luteal phase progesterone levels).
- **To avoid pregnancy**: If you persistently have short luteal phases, this can be very frustrating as you will have fewer days when you can safely have unprotected sex. Consider whether there is anything you could change – for example, if you are stressed, think about how best you can manage the stress.

Monophasic charts

In some cycles there may be no ovulation (anovulatory cycle) and therefore no temperature rise. The temperature stays at the lower level throughout the cycle, producing a monophasic chart (one level). The period may start at the expected time or it may be earlier or later than expected. Monophasic charts are common in adolescents and women approaching the menopause. They may also occur after childbirth, after stopping contraceptive injections, and at times of stress – such as serious illness or extreme weight loss. Severe stress may stop periods completely.

Figure 3.12 shows a monophasic chart with temperatures persistently on one level – this possibly indicates that there was no ovulation. The temperature may be quite flat or there may be wider day-to-day variations, but the key feature is that, overall, the temperatures are on one level.

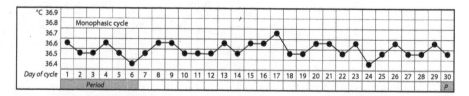

Figure 3.12 Monophasic chart (no temperature rise)

It sometimes helps to slide a ruler (or piece of paper) up from the bottom of the chart to determine whether there are one or two levels.

- **To conceive**: If you have three or more consecutive monophasic charts, talk to your doctor, who may wish to arrange blood tests including a progesterone test to confirm whether or not you are ovulating.
- **To avoid pregnancy**: If you notice any change from your normal biphasic pattern, contact your FAM practitioner. Monophasic charts can be difficult to interpret.

Fast facts

- The temperature rise normally occurs *after* ovulation. Temperature gives no advance warning of ovulation, so it is of limited value when trying to conceive.
- Temperature is of most value for avoiding pregnancy – when cross-checked with secretions, it confirms the *end* of the fertile time. The late infertile time is the most effective for avoiding pregnancy.
- The sustained rise in temperature indicates that ovulation is *likely* to have occurred but it is *not* definitive proof.

Combining temperature with secretions

When you combine temperature with secretions, consider each indicator on its own merit and then see how they correlate. Extend the shading on peak day upwards to see where peak occurs in relation to your temperature rise. Normally the temperature rise occurs just after peak day, but this can vary.

Figure 3.13 shows temperature and secretions on a combined chart. The first five days are the period, days 6 and 7 are dry. On day 8 there are moist, white, cloudy, sticky secretions so the fertile time has started. The secretions are wetter, slippery, transparent and stretchy from day 12 until day 14, with a distinct change back to dryness on day 15; so, day 14 is marked as peak (shaded column creating the 'chimney' effect). The

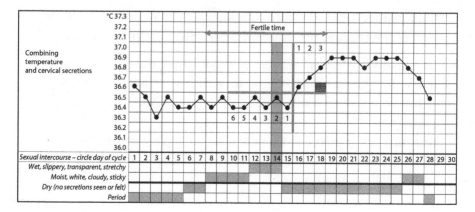

Figure 3.13 Combining temperature and secretions

first high temperature is on day 16 with the third high temperature on day 18. The third high temperature is at least 0.2 °C above the low temperatures. The horizontal arrow indicates the fertile time – from day 8 (first sign of secretions) until day 18 (third high temperature after peak day) inclusive.

- **To conceive**: The fertile time starts at the first sign of secretions and ends after the third high temperature past peak day.
- **To avoid pregnancy**: Secretions are a good cross-check with temperature for the end of the fertile time but there is still only one indicator at the start – this is where calendar-based calculations are of value (see Figure 4.1).

4 Cervix

Charting changes in the cervix is optional. You may not feel comfortable checking your cervix for personal, religious or cultural reasons. However, if you are keen to know your cervix better, it can be a really useful indicator.

There is no benefit to checking your cervix if you are planning pregnancy, but, if you are avoiding pregnancy, this gives valuable extra warning of approaching fertility. Cervical changes are particularly useful if you are struggling to observe secretions or if temperatures are not reliable (e.g. with shift work). Cervical changes are also useful if you plan to breastfeed for a long time or if you are approaching the menopause – times when ovulation may be delayed for many weeks.

Cervical changes through the cycle

Estrogen and progesterone cause subtle changes in the cervix. Just after a period, the cervix is low and easy to reach. It feels quite firm (rather like the tip of your nose) and the external os (cervical opening) will be closed. If you feel along the length of your cervix, it will be relatively long and tilted off-centre. As the estrogen levels increase, your cervix will rise higher, become softer (more like the texture of your bottom lip) and shorter in length (stubbier). It will be more centrally positioned (straighter), and the os will feel slightly open. After ovulation, under the influence of progesterone, the cervix changes back relatively quickly to its low, firm, closed, tilted position.

The most dramatic cervical change is when giving birth, at which time it dilates to 10 cm to form the birth passage. It returns to its non-pregnant state by six to 12 weeks after the birth, but it will forever remain slightly changed. If you are nulliparous (have never given birth), your cervical os will be small and round – rather like the mouth of a small fish; the os will feel tightly closed in its infertile state and relaxed enough to form a slight dimple in its fertile state. If you have given birth (parous), your cervical os will feel more slit-like, remaining slightly open at all times, but opening further at the fertile time – it may feel wide enough to admit your fingertip.

Figure 3.14 shows the changes in the cervix through the cycle (nulliparous women) with the cervix rising higher in the vagina, becoming softer and shorter in length at the fertile time. Note the dotted line which shows the relative height. It takes approximately one week to change from its lowest, firmest, closed position to its maximum height, softness and openness. After ovulation, it changes back within 24 hours to its low, firm, closed, tilted position.

Checking your cervix

Check your cervix at roughly the same time each day: preferably in the morning (e.g. at shower time). Make sure you have an empty bladder.

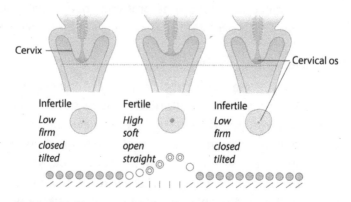

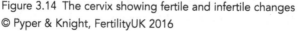

Figure 3.14 The cervix showing fertile and infertile changes
© Pyper & Knight, FertilityUK 2016

Start daily checks from the time your period ends. If you have very short cycles or long periods, you may need to start earlier.

1 Make sure your hands are clean with no long or broken fingernails.
2 Use the same position (either squatting or with one leg raised on the side of the bath or a chair)
3 Gently insert one or two fingers into your vagina and reach for your cervix. It feels rather like a smooth indented ball compared with the soft, ridged vaginal walls
4 Use a delicate fingertip touch to estimate the relative height (low or high in the vagina), texture (firm or soft), position (tilted or straight) and dilatation (closed or open)
5 If your cervix is hard to reach, try pushing down on the top of your uterus by pressing on your abdomen with the opposite hand, just above your pubic bone.

⚠ Monitoring secretions at the cervix

While checking your cervix, some secretions may come away on your finger(s). Secretions taken directly from the cervix provide an earlier warning compared with external observation, because it takes time for secretions to travel down the ridged vaginal walls. The most important thing is consistency in your approach: either check secretions internally or externally.

Recording cervical changes on the chart

Use the following symbols to record cervical changes:

- A solid black dot to represent a low, firm, closed cervix. A slanted line below to show the tilt – all signs of infertility
- An open circle to represent softness and an inner circle to represent an open os. A straight line below to show that the cervix is straight in position – all signs of fertility

Place the symbols in the box at a level which represents the relative height of the cervix (Figure 3.14 and Figure 4.2):

- The fertile time starts at the *first* sign of the cervix moving higher or becoming softer, more open or straighter.
- The fertile time ends when the cervix has returned to its low, firm, closed and tilted state and has remained so for *three full days*.

Few women will be able to detect all the changes, but, with time and patience, the cervix can be a valuable additional indicator. If you are just starting out with FAMs, it is often best to delay checking your cervix until you are more confident with identifying the other indicators.

- **To conceive**: The most fertile time is when the cervix is high, soft open and straight.
- **To avoid pregnancy**: The first change in the cervix helps to identify the start of the fertile time, but you need a cross-check of two indicators at the start and end of the fertile time (see above). Never rely on cervical changes alone.

⚠ Retroverted uterus

If your observations don't fit the description, you may have a retroverted uterus. The usual position is *anteverted* – the uterus slants forwards towards the pubic bone and the cervix projects downwards into the vagina. However, about one in five women have a *retroverted* uterus – the uterus slants backwards, pointing towards the small of the back, and the cervix points upwards slightly. The cervix may feel higher at the infertile time and lower at the fertile time, but the other characteristics are the same. In Figure 3.14, the symbols are shown rising at the fertile time, but with a retroverted uterus, they may form a U-shaped-curve.

A retroverted uterus is not a problem – it does not mean it will be more difficult to conceive.

Minor indicators

Cyclic changes such as abdominal pain, bloating, breast tenderness, skin changes and variations in mood and libido are *minor* indicators of fertility. Some changes are more marked around ovulation, while others are more marked premenstrually. These vary from woman to woman and from one cycle to the next.

'Ovulation' pain (mittelschmerz)

Ovulation pain may be felt as a cramp-like pain or dull ache on one side of your lower abdomen, typically lasting between 12 and 24 hours. The pain may radiate into your groin or vagina. The cause of the pain is unclear: it could be related to pressure from the distended follicle, or fluid from the ruptured follicle irritating the peritoneum (membrane lining the abdominal cavity), or it could be contractions of the fallopian tube as the egg passes along it. Ultrasound scans show that this pain coincides more closely with ovulation than any other minor indicators but its timing is still extremely varied. Pain does *not* confirm ovulation and being pain-free does not mean that there has been no ovulation. **Persistent or severe abdominal pain should always be promptly investigated** because it could indicate a serious condition such as appendicitis, an ovarian cyst or an ectopic pregnancy.

Abdominal bloating

Abdominal bloating is common. You may feel more bloated around the time of ovulation and/or around a period. You may notice appetite changes through your cycle, often craving carbs premenstrually.

Breast changes

You may notice a characteristic tenderness or tingling around your nipples at the time of ovulation, then fuller, heavier, painful breasts just before a period. Know what is normal for you – be breast aware (see Chapter 2).

Spotting or light bleeding

Bleeding between periods or bleeding after intercourse is not normal and should always be investigated to exclude infections such as chlamydia and gynaecological problems including cervical cancer. Make sure your cervical screening is up-to-date and tell your doctor if you notice any unusual bleeding including bleeding between periods or after sex. In very rare cases, a few spots of blood or blood-tinged secretions close to peak day may be hormone-related, but this always requires investigation.

It is common to have pink/brown spotting for up to two days before the bright-red period bleeding starts, but, if you are trying to conceive and you consistently have *more than* two days of spotting, this may indicate a problem with implantation. Prolonged premenstrual spotting may be a sign of hormonal changes (lower levels of progesterone) or gynaecological conditions such as polyps (benign growths in the uterus or cervix), endometriosis, adenomyosis or fibroids which can cause heavy and painful periods.

Mood and libido

Many women notice cyclic changes in mood and libido (sex drive). Some have more energy, a higher sex drive and a greater sense of wellbeing approaching ovulation (when estrogen is dominant), but a more depressed mood with tiredness, irritability and a low sex drive premenstrually (when progesterone is dominant). Conversely, some women feel more like sex premenstrually. Mood and libido can be affected by hormones, but other physical and psychological factors are often involved. If you experience severe mood changes, talk to your doctor because extreme forms of premenstrual syndrome (PMS) can be debilitating and may require medication.

Recording minor indicators on the chart

Record minor indicators on your chart by the appropriate day or in the comments box. It may be interesting to see how symptoms such as abdominal pain correlate with peak day or the temperature rise, but **these changes should never be relied on.**

Disturbances affecting the chart

Note any disturbance or change from routine on your chart. Some disturbances affect specific indicators, while others (such as stress) may cause more generalized cycle disturbance.

Disturbances affecting temperature

A number of disturbances affect resting temperature causing erratic readings – some occur more frequently than others.

Checklist of factors which may affect resting temperature

- Alcohol
- Late night, disrupted sleep, lie-in
- Shift work: late/early shifts and particularly night shifts
- Holidays, travel: particularly long-haul air travel and crossing time zones
- Daylight saving/changing the clocks
- Anxiety and stress
- Illness: acute or chronic
- Some bought or prescribed drugs (including painkillers)
- Some herbal preparations

A single disturbed reading might result in a temperature spike (see above), but if there is a disturbance on consecutive days this may cause more prolonged disruption. Use a coloured pen to record disturbed readings, giving an explanation for the disturbance (if known) either by the affected temperature(s) or in the comments box.

Weekend disturbances

If you normally take your temperature when your alarm goes off from Monday to Friday, but you have a lie-in on Saturday and Sunday morning – this is likely to produce two consecutive raised temperatures (see Figure 4.4) – these must *not* be confused with the ovulation rise. A weekend disturbance often includes a combination of alcohol, a later evening meal, a late night and possibly a lie-in. To identify weekend disturbances more easily, record the days of the week across the top of the chart and highlight the weekends.

Shift work

Shift work can be challenging. Your chart may show signs of stress including changes in cycle length, a delayed or absent temperature rise and short luteal phases. If you work early and late shifts, you may be able to adjust your temperature readings to compensate for the variations in the time you take your temperature (see above). If you work night shifts, you may need to experiment a little. Most women get a consistent reading by taking their temperature after their longest sleep, but the alternative is to continue taking your temperature at your usual target time regardless of how it relates to sleep.

Changing the clocks: daylight saving

Disturbances such as changing the clocks can disrupt the temperature for several days. In spring, when the clocks go forward, this has the same effect as taking your temperature an hour earlier – so temperatures may be slightly lower; in the autumn, when the clocks go back, this has the same effect as taking it an hour later – so your temperatures may be slightly higher. If the clocks change when you are expecting your temperature rise, cross-check your other indicators carefully, although you may not be able to interpret your chart.

Illness and drugs

Illness such as a vague sore throat tends to produce only mildly raised temperatures, but some ill-health conditions may result in a fever with temperatures much higher than normal (often going off the top of the fertility chart). Drugs such as paracetamol reduce temperature so you may get a lower reading than normal if you have taken painkillers less than four hours before you take your temperature.

With experience, you should be able to make adjustments for common disturbances, but when disturbances occur randomly, this can be confusing. You will find more information on factors affecting the cycle including crossing time zones in *The Complete Guide to Fertility Awareness* (see Resources). **Remember, disturbed readings may make it impossible to interpret your chart.**

Difficulties monitoring cervical secretions

It takes time to learn to distinguish changes in cervical secretions – the pattern can vary and some external factors cause confusion. Consider the following:

- **First cycle**: It helps if you avoid intercourse completely when you start charting so you can recognize your own pattern of secretions without confusion from other fluids.
- **Secretions just before a period**: It is common to notice secretions (sometimes clear wet secretions) just before your period starts – this is related to falling progesterone levels which allow a brief rise in estrogen. These are not fertile secretions – they can be disregarded.
- **Short cycles**: If you have short cycles, you may not have any dry days. You may notice sticky or wet, stretchy secretions towards the end of your period or immediately afterwards, indicating that your fertile time has started.
- **Long cycles**: If you have long cycles, you may have many dry days following your period or an interrupted pattern of secretions (see below).
- **Variations in quantity and quality**: The amount and quality of secretions will vary. It is often easier to detect secretions at the vulva after exercise, after a bowel movement, or by bearing down slightly.
- **Little or no wetter secretions**: The quantity and quality of secretions decrease with age. Older women may notice only small amounts (if any) of the transparent, wet secretions due to lower estrogen levels. Similarly, women who are underweight with little body fat may have reduced estrogen stores and less of the wetter secretions.
- **Persistent secretions**: If you have persistent secretions and rarely (or never) have any dry days, you may have a cervical ectropion – a

harmless condition of the cervix in which the lining of the cervical canal protrudes onto the outer part of the cervix. This is sometimes noticed during cervical screening. If you are troubled by excessive secretions, talk to your doctor.

- **Interrupted pattern of secretions**: The secretions may start off sticky and white, stop for a few days and then restart sticky and white, building up to wetter, slippery secretions. The fertile time starts at the *first* sign of secretions and continues until a cross-check of temperature and secretions confirms the end of the fertile time. This commonly occurs in longer cycles, at times of stress and with conditions such as polycystic ovary syndrome (PCOS).

- **Double peak**: You can have more than one peak day. The secretions build up normally to peak day, after which you notice a distinct change back to less fertile characteristics; however, then the wetter, slippery secretions return and you have a second peak. The fertile time starts at the *first sign* of secretions and continues until a cross-check of temperature and secretions confirms the end of the fertile time (after the second peak). In some cases, there may even be a third peak. Multiple peaks commonly occur at times of illness or stress and with PCOS.

- **Pelvic floor exercises**: Practising pelvic floor (Kegel) exercises helps to increase the sensation at the vulva. To identify the relevant muscles: try to stop a flow of urine mid-stream, or insert one or two fingers into your vagina and alternately contract and relax the muscles, gripping and releasing your fingers. If there are no secretions, the vaginal lips feel dry – a feeling of 'nothingness'. If you have sticky secretions, the lips feel sticky as they separate, and if you have slippery secretions, the lips slide apart smoothly.

- **Confusion with other fluids**: It is easy to get confused by other bodily fluids. Arousal fluid is transparent and slippery but, unlike cervical secretions, it has no stretch. Seminal fluid is sticky and slightly rubbery. It breaks easily and dries more quickly than egg-white-type cervical secretions. Vaginal lubricants are usually transparent and give a lubricative sensation so they could be confused with highly fertile cervical secretions; however, you will know if you have used lube. If you use spermicide with a diaphragm/cap, check its colour, texture and odour – with experience you should be able to tell the difference between spermicide and cervical secretions.

- **Skin sensitivity and allergic reactions**: Vulval skin is delicate. Avoid perfumed or coloured soaps and bath products – use baby soap or non-allergic bath products. Avoid talcum powders, vaginal deodorants and douches as these may affect the pH balance of the vagina and destroy the normal lactic-acid-producing bacteria which keep the vagina healthy.
- **Reducing your risk of infections**: A warm, moist environment is a perfect breeding ground for bugs, so pay attention to your personal hygiene. Avoid nylon underwear, tights and restrictive clothing – breathable cotton pants are cooler and more absorbent. Avoid thongs because they provide a direct route for infections to pass from the rectum to the vagina and urethra, increasing your risk of recurrent thrush or cystitis. If you use tampons, use the appropriate absorbency and avoid tampons on days of light bleeding because they can be drying and disrupt the normal vaginal flora. Avoid unnecessary use of sanitary pads and mini-pads as they absorb natural vaginal secretions and can cause chafing and sometimes a reactive discharge. **Report abnormal discharges to your doctor promptly**.
- **Illness or stress**: Illness or stress can delay or suppress ovulation and consequently disrupt the normal pattern of secretions. You may notice persistent dryness, an interrupted pattern of secretions, a double peak or a shorter interval from peak day to the next period.
- **Effect of drugs**: Some drugs such as antihistamines (e.g. for hay fever) may dry up cervical secretions. Other drugs such as guaifenesin (also known as glyceryl guaiacolate) in expectorant cough mixture may increase cervical secretions. Check any medicines you buy with a pharmacist before you take them, especially if you are trying to conceive.

Test kits, monitors, gadgets and apps

It would be nice to think that technology could provide a shortcut to finding the fertile time – so what about all the widely available kits, gadgets and apps? The real issue here is that there are few controls on these technologies – they can be marketed without rigorous testing and there is little reliable evidence about their effectiveness under real-life conditions. One of the biggest problems for technologies to overcome is cycle disturbances. If you understand your own fertility and the factors that disturb your cycles, you may be able to use technology intelligently, but don't believe it has the answer.

Ovulation predictor kits

Ovulation predictor kits (OPKs) do just as their name implies – they predict when ovulation is likely to occur. You test your urine on specific days to detect LH (luteinizing hormone) which surges 24–36 hours before ovulation. The LH surge may help to define the two most fertile days, but it does not define the full fertile time. Some kits analyse both LH and estrogen so they typically identify four fertile days. OPKs are designed for *planning* pregnancy. If you get a positive result, it shows that you have had an LH surge (which usually triggers ovulation) but it does not prove that you have released an egg. If you have a hormone imbalance such as polycystic ovarian syndrome (PCOS) with raised LH levels, these kits can give false readings. OPKs do *not* give sufficient warning for avoiding pregnancy.

Fertility monitors

A fertility monitor consists of a handheld computer and disposable urine test sticks which measure estrogen and LH. Two monitors, Clearblue and Persona, are the result of years of scientific research. As they work directly on the ovarian hormones, they have a high degree of accuracy provided they are used according to the manufacturer's instructions. The main disadvantage is their high cost, with ongoing costs for test sticks.

Clearblue fertility monitor

The Clearblue fertility monitor is aimed at women who are planning pregnancy. It requires cycles to be in the range of 21–42 days, and typically identifies six fertile days. Clearblue predicts days of low, high and peak fertility using a series of bars.

Persona (Clearblue contraceptive monitor)

Persona is aimed at women who are avoiding pregnancy. It can be used by women with cycles ranging from 23 to 35 days. It gives a red light for fertile days and a green light for infertile days. Some women combine Persona with charting (see Figure 4.4). Persona is available in the UK, but in the USA and other parts of Europe this device is known as the Clearblue contraceptive monitor. When used alone, Persona is about 94 per cent effective – this means that, if 100 women use Persona correctly for one year, six women would be expected to become pregnant.

Computerized thermometers

Some devices combine an electronic thermometer with a small computer which analyses temperature and cycle length. Some computerized thermometers allow you to enter information about secretions, hormone tests and intercourse. More research is needed before these devices can be recommended for avoiding pregnancy. There is no reliable evidence to support claims made for devices which include a sex-selection feature.

Some devices measure body temperature through an adhesive patch which is worn continuously, or a vaginal probe or bracelet worn overnight; a sensor then analyses the temperatures to show days with the highest chance of pregnancy. There is currently no evidence to suggest that these expensive continuous monitoring devices offer any advantage over simple digital thermometers combined with knowledge about secretions.

Saliva testing kits

Saliva testing kits use a plastic mini-microscope to detect a characteristic ferning pattern in saliva as a sign of ovulation. Research shows these are unreliable. One study found the ferning pattern in post-menopausal women and in men! The use of these kits is strongly discouraged.

Fertility apps

Fertility apps (sometimes referred to as period trackers) offer a convenient way to record and store information about menstrual cycles, but with over 1,000 apps on the market it is almost impossible to work out which is the most suitable. Some apps simply track period dates, but others allow you to enter information about different fertility indicators.

Research shows that the vast majority of apps contain misleading health information and are inaccurate. The most reliable apps are not necessarily the ones which have the most appealing user interface or the most convincing marketing hype. Many apps provide a computerized chart interpretation, some allow you to disable this feature and make your own interpretation, and some allow you to submit charts to online forums. It is important to recognize that this market is unregulated so there is no quality assurance. There are also concerns about privacy and security. This concern has been voiced at the highest levels. In July 2022, the White House warned individuals who live in states where abortion has become illegal to be very careful about the use of period trackers over fears that their data could be used against them in future criminal cases.

Only enter personal information that you are comfortable to share with others – remember, you are not only sharing your information (which includes sensitive information about how often you have sex), but you are also sharing your partner's information – do you have their consent?

It is fine to use a fertility app purely for interest or to help you plan pregnancy but, with the currently available evidence, fertility apps *cannot* be recommended for avoiding pregnancy.

4

Using fertility awareness methods to avoid pregnancy

This chapter is aimed at women of normal fertility who wish to avoid pregnancy. The following three chapters cover specific circumstances: after hormonal contraception, after childbirth and approaching the menopause. FAMs are highly effective, provided women are properly taught, use a combination of indicators and follow the appropriate guidelines. The information is intended to supplement teaching from an accredited practitioner (see the list of organizations teaching FAMs in Resources).

Identifying the start of the fertile time

You will by now be familiar with the different indicators. If pregnancy is to be avoided, the indicators need to be combined in a way that provides the most conservative (safest) interpretation. The earliest warning of the fertile time usually comes from a calculation based on past cycle lengths. This normally gives a day or two extra warning compared with the first change in secretions or cervix.

Calculations to identify the start of the fertile time

First, consider which calculation is right for you based on your cycle length. This is no time for guesswork: 'about 28 days' is not good enough – you need precise dates from your diary or an app. If you have not been recording cycle lengths – start now. If you have a record of your last 12 cycle lengths, start using the S minus 20 rule (Chapter 3 and below). If you have no written record, start with the Day 6 rule (below).

Day 6 rule

First fertile day is day 6. You can have unprotected intercourse up until the end of day 5, but, from day 6 onwards, you must abstain or use a barrier method.

The day 6 rule has some provisos:

- *Cycle 1*: Learning cycle only – avoid all unprotected intercourse.
- *Cycles 2 and 3*: To establish whether you have short cycles: you cannot rely on this yet.
- *Cycles 4–12*:
  - If your first three cycles were 26 days or longer, it is now safe to have unprotected intercourse up until the end of day 5.
  - If your first three cycles were *shorter* than 26 days, the Day 6 rule will not work for you. You would be at risk of pregnancy early in your cycle, so should restrict unprotected intercourse to the late infertile time
- *Cycle 13 onwards*: You should now have an accurate record of your past 12 cycle lengths so you can apply the S minus 20 rule.

S minus 20 rule

Consider the last 12 cycle lengths, find the shortest (S) and subtract 20 to find your first fertile day.

S minus 20 = first fertile day

For example: Suppose your last 12 cycles were 27, 31, 29, 28, 30, 29, 27, 27, 30, 29, 27 and 28 days, your shortest cycle is 27 days; 27 – 20 = 7, so day 7 is your first fertile day. You can have unprotected intercourse from the start of your period up until the end of day 6.

Update your calculation at the end of each cycle based on your 12 *most recent* cycle lengths.

> ### Earliest temperature rise minus 7 rule
>
> Once you have charted temperatures for 12 cycles, you can get an even more precise marker of the start of your fertile time. This supersedes the S minus 20 and Day 6 rules. From your 12 most recent cycles, identify the *earliest* temperature rise and subtract seven to identify the first fertile day.
>
> **Earliest temperature rise minus 7 = first fertile day**
>
> *For example*: Suppose in your last 12 cycles, your first high temperature occurred on days 15, 17, 16, 15, 16, 16, 15, 16, 18, 17, 16 and 15, respectively, and your earliest rise was on day 15. Quick sum: 15 – 7 = 8. Your first fertile day would therefore be day 8 (you can have unprotected intercourse up until the end of day 7). If you have an earlier temperature rise in a subsequent cycle, adjust the calculation accordingly – it is always based on the 12 *most recent* cycles.

Figure 4.1 shows a flow diagram of the different calculations. If you continue to have unprotected intercourse after the day given by your calculation, your risk of pregnancy increases significantly.

'Stop bar'

It is helpful to put a short vertical line – a 'stop bar' – on your chart to indicate the start of the fertile time (Figure 4.3). Do this at the beginning of your period when you have updated your calculation. The stop bar is a reminder that there should be no unprotected sex after the bar.

Earliest sign of change

Calculations usually give the earliest indication of the fertile time, but watch for any change from dryness, because occasionally secretions start before the day given by the calculation. Similarly, cervical changes occasionally give the earliest warning. **The fertile time starts on the day identified by the calculation, the first sign of secretions, or the first change in the cervix, whichever occurs first.**

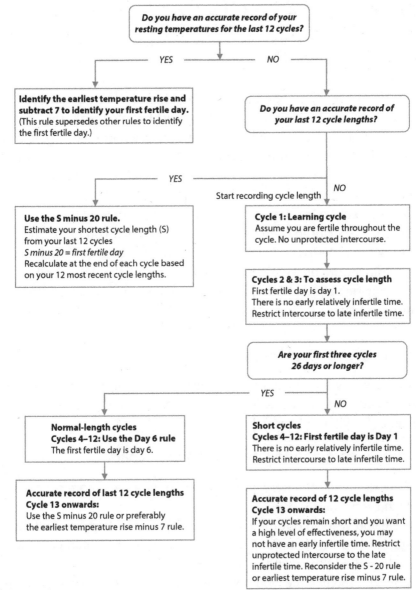

Do you have an accurate record of your resting temperatures for the last 12 cycles?

YES — NO

Identify the earliest temperature rise and subtract 7 to identify your first fertile day.
(This rule supersedes other rules to identify the first fertile day.)

Do you have an accurate record of your last 12 cycle lengths?

YES — NO

Start recording cycle length

Use the S minus 20 rule.
Estimate your shortest cycle length (S) from your last 12 cycles
S minus 20 = first fertile day
Recalculate at the end of each cycle based on your 12 most recent cycle lengths.

Cycle 1: Learning cycle
Assume you are fertile throughout the cycle. No unprotected intercourse.

Cycles 2 & 3: To assess cycle length
First fertile day is day 1.
There is no early relatively infertile time.
Restrict intercourse to late infertile time.

Are your first three cycles 26 days or longer?

YES — NO

Normal-length cycles
Cycles 4–12: Use the Day 6 rule
The first fertile day is day 6.

Short cycles
Cycles 4–12: First fertile day is Day 1
There is no early relatively infertile time.
Restrict intercourse to late infertile time.

Accurate record of last 12 cycle lengths
Cycle 13 onwards:
Use the S minus 20 rule or preferably the earliest temperature rise minus 7 rule.

Accurate record of 12 cycle lengths
Cycle 13 onwards:
If your cycles remain short and you want a high level of effectiveness, you may not have an early infertile time. Restrict unprotected intercourse to the late infertile time. Reconsider the S - 20 rule or earliest temperature rise minus 7 rule.

Notes:
1. Draw a short vertical 'stop bar' to show the first fertile day based on the relevant calculation.
2. A calculation generally gives the earliest indication of the first fertile day (start of the fertile time); however, always be vigilant for any change in cervical secretions and/or cervical changes prior to the day given by your calculation. The fertile time starts at the earliest sign of change – whether from secretions, cervix or the calculation.

Figure 4.1 Calculations to identify the start of the fertile time

Identifying the end of the fertile time

The two key indicators used to identify the end of the fertile time are the temperature and secretions. Use the 3 over 6 rule (see Chapter 3) to identify three high temperatures above the previous six low-phase temperatures (remembering that the third high temperature must be at least 0.2 °C). All the high temperatures must be after peak day. The fertile time ends after the third high temperature past peak day. It is safe to resume intercourse from the evening of the third high temperature after peak day. The late infertile time lasts until the start of the next period – it is the most effective for avoiding pregnancy.

If you check your cervix, there is no need to wait until it has returned to its low, firm, closed state for three days, provided you have three high temperatures after peak day. However, there may be times when either your temperature or secretions may be less reliable and the cervical check may be helpful. With time and experience, you will learn to use your most reliable indicator.

Interpreting your chart

Always use a systematic approach when interpreting your chart to make sure you consider all the available information. Follow this step-by-step guide.

Step-by-step guide to interpreting your chart

- Consider what number chart you are on (you gain more experience with every chart).
- Have you worked out the most appropriate calculation to find the start of your fertile time? Recalculate this at the beginning of a new cycle and add the stop-bar reminder.
- Consider the first day you notice secretions – if this occurs before the day designated by the calculation, then this marks the start of your fertile time.
- Find your peak day – ensure it is the *last* day of wetter, transparent, stretchy secretions. Extend the shading upwards to the top of the temperature graph (make sure the day after peak was marked in a lower box).

- Look at the whole temperature graph – is it on one or two levels? Try placing a ruler or sheet of paper across all the temperatures to get an overall impression before looking at the details.
- Circle any temperature spikes – remember that a spike is a *single* temperature which is at least 0.2 °C above the one on both sides.
- Identify the relevant temperatures for the 3 over 6 rule. Draw your horizontal coverline on the line *immediately* above the highest of the low-phase temperatures; then draw a vertical line on the line which divides the low- and high-phase temperatures (forming a cross). Add hatching to the square above the coverline on the day of the third high temperature to make sure it is at least 0.2 °C (the dot cannot be in the hatched square). If the third high temperature is not at least 0.2 °C, wait for a fourth high temperature which just needs to be above the coverline. Starting at the point the cross intersects, number the high-phase temperatures 1, 2, 3 (above the relevant temperatures) and the low-phase temperatures 1, 2, 3, 4, 5, 6 (in reverse order) beneath the relevant temperatures.
- Consider whether there are any temperature spikes among the six low-phase temperatures – remember you can safely ignore one spike, but if there is more than one spike you cannot interpret the chart.
- Consider whether any of the three high temperatures were disturbed – make sure that there are three *undisturbed* high temperatures.
- Now notice how your peak day fits with your temperatures. All of your high temperatures must be after peak day, so you may need to recount your high temperatures to make sure that you have three high temperatures after peak – they must be to the right of the 'chimney'. If you need to make a correction, write 1, 2, 3 boldly in red pen to show the three high temperatures after peak day.
- If you are recording cervical changes, check how your observations compare with your temperature and secretions. If you notice a change in your cervix early in your cycle before the day designated by your calculation and before any secretions, then regard the first change in your cervix as the start of your fertile time. Provided you have three high temperatures after peak day, there is no need to wait for your cervix to be low, firm and closed for three days to determine the end of your fertile time.

- Have you considered the impact of any disturbances – e.g. alcohol, medication?
- Can you apply the guidelines correctly?
- Add a horizontal arrow to show the start and end of the fertile time (using the safest interpretation).

Combining the indicators of fertility

To avoid pregnancy, ensure that you cross-check at least two indicators at the start and end of the fertile time. The following example charts show how to use the most conservative estimate to give the safest interpretation.

Example charts

The chart shown in Figure 4.2 is from a new user charting her third cycle. She has set her stop bar at day 6 using the Day 6 rule. The first cervical change is on day 8 which correlates with the first sign of secretions. Peak is on day 15. The first high temperature is on day 17. By day 19, there are three high temperatures after peak and the third high temperature is at least 0.2 °C. There is a temperature spike on days 5 and 13 (circled). There is only one spike in the six low temperatures, so it can safely be ignored. Note the way the cervix changes relatively slowly from day 8 onwards to reach its position of maximum height and openness, but it reverts more rapidly to its infertile state between days 15 and 17. The fertile time lasts from day 6 to 19 inclusive.

The chart shown in Figure 4.3 combines the S minus 20 rule with secretions, cervix and temperature. This is a 29-day cycle. The shortest cycle is 28 days so the stop bar is set at day 8. The first cervical change is on day 9 and the first secretions noted on day 10. The fertile time started on day 8 despite the individual still feeling dry and the cervix being low, firm and closed. Peak is on day 15, the same day as the temperature rise. Although by day 17 there are three high temperatures above the six low-phase temperatures (and the third temperature is at least 0.2 °C), the woman must wait another day until there are three high temperatures after peak day. The fertile time lasts from day 8 until day 18. By day 18, the cervix has been low, firm and closed for three days, but it is not necessary to wait for this, provided there has been a double check of temperature and secretions.

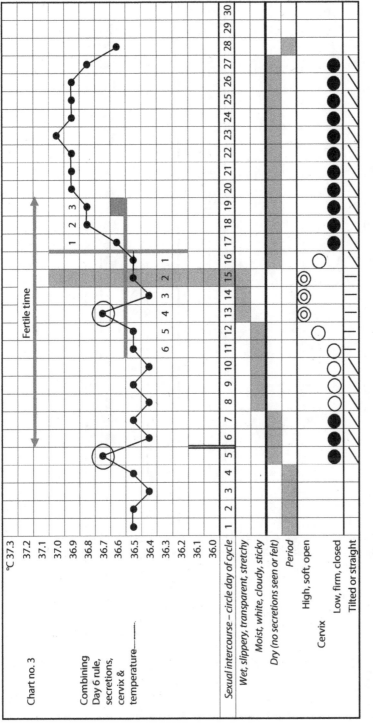

Figure 4.2 Combining Day 6 rule, secretions, cervix and temperature

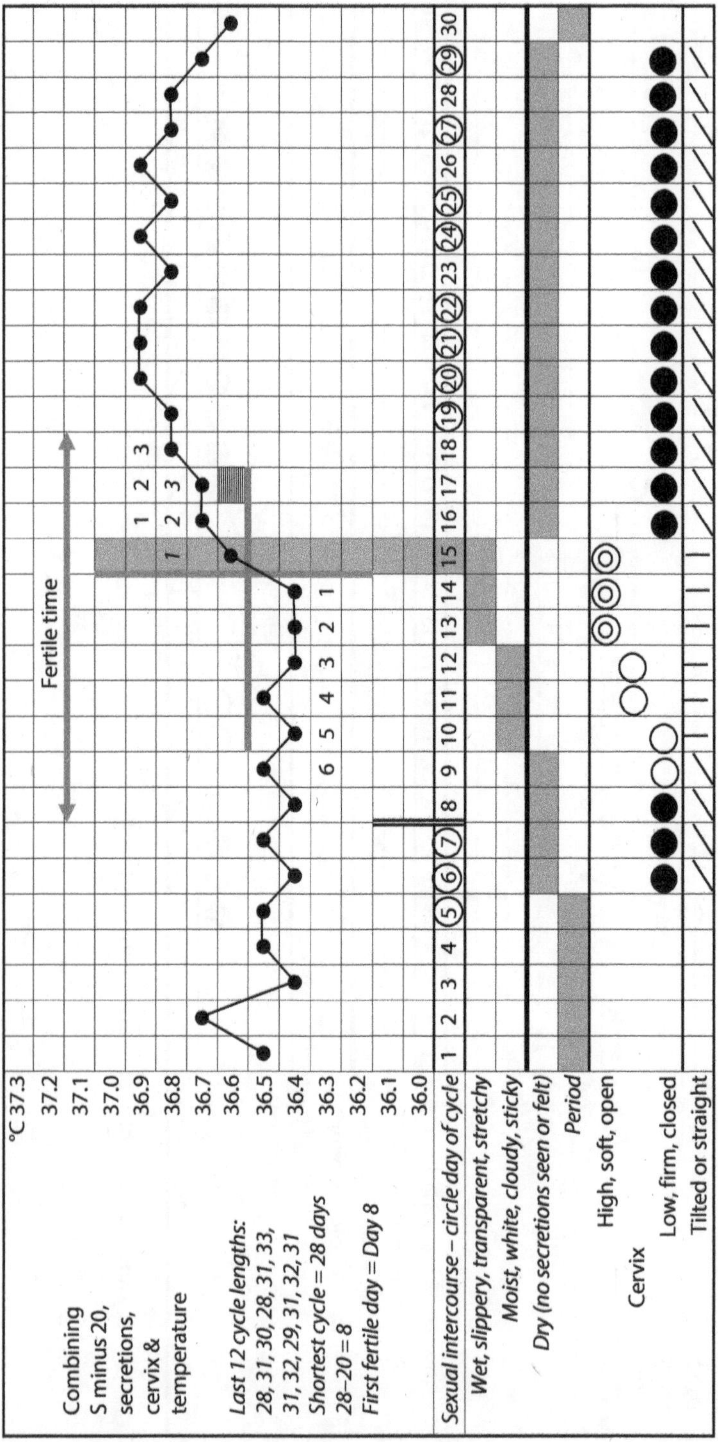

Figure 4.3 Combining S minus 20 calculation, secretions, cervix and temperature

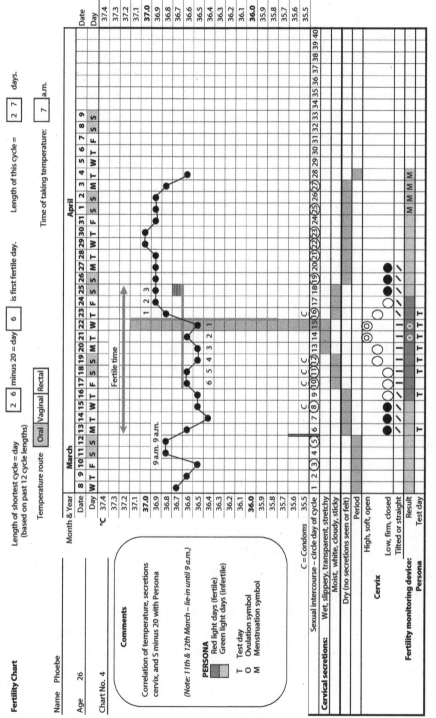

Figure 4.4 Combining all indicators with a fertility monitor

Choosing your combination of indicators

The first fertile day is usually identified by a combination of a calculation and secretions, and the last fertile day by three high temperatures after peak. It is possible to use a different combination of indicators, but the effectiveness of these approaches remains unknown. For example, at times when temperature may not be reliable (such as night shifts), some women rely on cervical changes combined with secretions. The fertile time would then start at the first change in cervix, the first secretions, or the calendar calculation, whichever occurs *earlier*, and the fertile time would end on the fourth evening after peak day or the third day of a low, firm, closed cervix, whichever occurs *later*. An experienced practitioner will help you to find the indicators that work best for you.

Some women combine their observations with a home kit (see Chapter 3). Figure 4.4 shows how Phoebe combines her observations with a fertility monitor. This is a 27-day cycle. The shortest cycle is 26 days, so her first fertile day is day 6. The monitor does not give the first red light (fertile) until day 9 (first day of cervical change and the day before secretions start). The last fertile day is day 18 (three high temperatures after peak). Persona gives a green light (infertile) again on day 18. The 'O' symbols (LH surge days) on days 14 and 15 correlate closely with peak and the days when the cervix is high, soft and open. 'C' on the chart indicates use of condoms during the fertile time. The monitor helps to increase Phoebe's confidence in her own observations.

Guidelines to avoid pregnancy through normal fertility

At the start of each cycle, ask yourself: was there a temperature rise in my last cycle?

If there was a temperature rise ten to 16 days before your bleed, this is a 'true period' and the guidelines can be applied.

If there was no temperature rise, the bleeding could be associated with ovulation. Assume you are fertile until you can confidently confirm the end of the fertile time.

First cycle

This a learning cycle only. No unprotected intercourse this cycle.

Second and subsequent cycles

Identifying the start of the fertile time (first fertile day)

The first fertile day is identified by:

- Calculation: S minus 20, Day 6, or Earliest temperature rise minus 7 – see Chapter 4 and Figure 4.1
- Secretions: First sign of *any* secretions (first change from dryness)
- Cervix: First sign of change from a low, firm, closed, tilted cervix

The first fertile day is the day shown by the *earliest* indicator.

Identifying the end of the fertile time (last fertile day)

The last fertile day is confirmed by:

- Temperature: evening of the third high temperature, provided that:
  - There are at least six low temperatures;
  - There are three consecutive undisturbed high temperatures;
  - The third high temperature is at least 0.2 °C above the six low temperatures (if not, wait for a fourth high temperature which just needs to be above the coverline).
- Cervical secretions: The three high temperatures must be after peak day.
- Cervix: the cervix should be low, firm, closed and tilted for three days.

If temperature and secretions correlate, there is no need to wait for the cervix to be closed for three days.

Building up your charting experience

It takes time to build up your confidence in FAMs. As a new user, it is important to record your indicators every day to get into the habit of charting and to see a pattern. With the experience of one year's charts, you will have had time to build up a record of your cycle length, normal pattern of secretions, usual coverline and your earliest temperature rise – this allows you to introduce more personalized calculations. You may be able to increase the number of days when you can have unprotected sex, yet still have a highly effective method. After one year, you are likely to have observed the effects of common disturbances such as alcohol, disrupted sleep, holidays, stress, illness and medication – you are now considered an experienced user.

Although many women enjoy the discipline of daily charting, some prefer to limit the number of days when charting is required. This is fine, provided you have enough information to make a safe interpretation. For example, provided your last 12 cycles have all been 26 days or longer, there is no need to take your temperature during your period, begin recording when your calculation indicates the start of the fertile time. Then take your temperature consistently every morning until the end of the fertile time. If you have short cycles, start recording temperatures from day 1 to ensure you have enough readings. Once you have confirmed that the fertile time has ended, you can discontinue charting until your next period starts.

Figure 4.5 shows a chart recorded by Mandy, an experienced user – this is her twenty-first chart. Day 7 is her first fertile day based on the earliest temperature rise minus 7 rule. She therefore starts recording temperatures on day 7 and continues until she is confident that the fertile time is over. Her third high temperature is only 0.1 °C above the low readings, so she waits for the fourth reading to make sure that it is above the coverline. She has recorded her secretions from the start of her cycle, but she stops once she has observed peak day and made sure that all her high temperatures are after peak. She has recorded cervical changes for the duration of her fertile time to confirm her other observations. She has one temperature spike on day 12 which seems to be related to alcohol the night before. She noted abdominal pain on her peak day and some premenstrual breast symptoms. Mandy has sufficient information to interpret her chart with confidence.

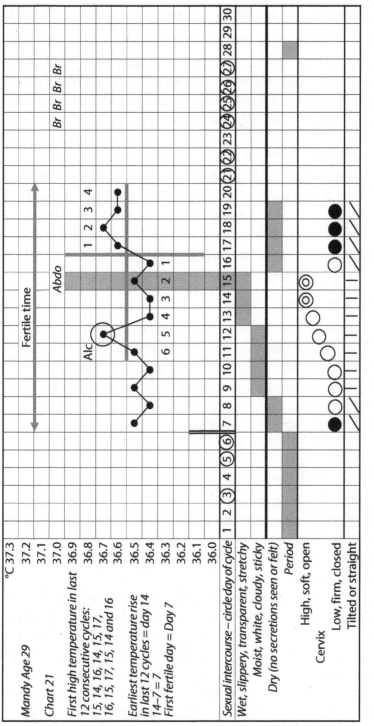

Figure 4.5 Experienced user who only charts on the essential days

Effectiveness of fertility awareness methods (FAMs)

When motivated couples are taught by accredited FAM practitioners to use a combination of indicators, and use the guidelines consistently, FAMs are up to 99 per cent effective. This means that about one woman in 100 will conceive in a year if using the method correctly. If FAMs are not used according to instructions, more women will get pregnant.

Early versus late infertile times

The late infertile time (post-ovulatory) provides maximum effectiveness, so if you have a very strong need to avoid pregnancy, you could restrict intercourse to the late infertile time. The early infertile time (pre-ovulatory) is only ever *relatively* infertile because there is always a possibility that you might have your shortest cycle ever, or a batch of super-sperm could survive longer than expected.

Sex during the fertile time

The effectiveness of FAMs relies on your ability to accurately identify the signs of fertility, and then to either abstain from intercourse (natural family planning) or use a barrier method during the fertile time. The choice is a personal one: some couples choose to abstain completely during the fertile time for personal or religious reasons, whilst others are open to the use of barrier methods (or withdrawal) either regularly or occasionally.

Natural family planning with abstinence

If you choose to abstain during the fertile time, you will be faced with times when you must avoid intercourse and all genital contact. The average time of abstinence for women of normal fertility is around ten days each cycle, but it can be longer at times of uncertainty or hormonal change.

The term abstinence has negative connotations, yet many couples report that abstinence (waiting) enhances their sexual relationship. Some couples avoid all forms of sexual activity during the fertile time, whilst others use 'outercourse' – different forms of sex play including oral sex, mutual masturbation, massage, body rubbing, fantasy and sex toys. Outercourse is almost 100 per cent effective against pregnancy provided that the man does not ejaculate near the woman's vulva.

It is important to be able to talk openly with your partner about your sexual needs and how you both feel about times of abstinence. You should be able to discuss this freely with your FAM practitioner.

FAMs with barrier methods

The use of barrier methods during the fertile time can work well. It is important to use a reliable method (male or female condom, or diaphragm/cap) consistently and carefully – your local contraception and sexual health clinic can provide barrier methods and instructions for use.

If you use barriers during the fertile time, you must continue to chart your cycles meticulously and use your chosen barrier for any intercourse during the fertile time. If you use a diaphragm with spermicide, you need to be able to distinguish between spermicide and secretions – see Chapter 3.

FAMs combined with barriers can be highly effective provided you use your knowledge intelligently. Many couples use barriers on the days they consider are 'low risk' at the margins of the fertile time, then avoid intercourse completely on 'high risk' days (the few days with highly fertile-type secretions). Note that effectiveness figures for barrier methods are based on couples who use the method throughout the menstrual cycle. If you use a barrier method on a day you recognize is highly fertile, and the barrier fails, there is a significant chance of pregnancy.

5

Using fertility awareness methods after hormonal contraception

Hormonal contraception contains small amounts of synthetic hormone(s) which inhibit natural hormone production. Some methods contain two hormones – estrogen and progestogen (synthetic form of progesterone); others contain just progestogen. The hormones are delivered in a variety of ways: pills, patches, vaginal rings, injections, implants and intrauterine systems (IUS). Hormonal methods prevent pregnancy by disrupting the normal menstrual cycle. Most methods have a dual action: they prevent ovulation and block sperm penetration through the cervical canal; some methods rely purely on the blocking effect at the cervix and ovulation continues to occur. While using hormonal contraception, the bleeding is not a proper period – it is a hormone 'withdrawal' bleed. Withdrawal bleeds are usually light, pain-free and pinkish or dark red/brown in colour – they may be regular or irregular. With the implant or injection, you may not have any vaginal bleeding.

When you stop the pill, patch, ring, implant or IUS, fertility normally returns very quickly. Sometimes ovulation can be delayed and periods can be irregular for a few cycles, but generally fertility returns immediately. The only hormonal method where there is commonly a longer delay is the contraceptive injection – it can take up to a year or more for normal fertility to return.

Be ready to start your new method *immediately* after stopping the hormonal method. If you are switching to FAMs, make sure you have found a practitioner and you are ready to start charting. The indicators of fertility can be confusing for a while making it more difficult to interpret charts. If you are avoiding pregnancy, you need to either use a barrier method consistently or abstain from sex completely until you can confidently identify your fertile time. If you are coming off hormonal contraception to conceive, it is safe to start trying immediately (see Chapter 8).

What to expect after stopping hormonal contraception

After stopping any hormonal method, your cycles may be disturbed for a while – you may notice variations in your bleeding pattern, cycle length, temperature or secretions.

Changes in vaginal bleeding

As your normal periods resume, they are likely to be heavier and brighter red with more painful cramps – this is due to the effect of the progesterone (following ovulation) thickening the endometrium. It is only considered a 'true period' if there has been a temperature rise ten to 16 days earlier. Start a new chart at the start of a true period. If you get any bleeding without a preceding temperature rise, it could be due to hormonal fluctuations associated with ovulation – the bleeding should be regarded as a sign of fertility. Continue on the same chart (joining two together if needed) until you get a true period.

ⓘ Recognizing a 'true period'

- A 'true period' is preceded by a temperature rise ten to 16 days earlier.
- Any bleeding not defined as a true period is potentially fertile.

Variations in cycle length

Anticipate that your cycles will not be regular at first. They may not be the same length as before you started hormonal contraception. The first few cycles can be particularly variable, so you should not use a fertility monitor or any device that makes predictions based on cycle length for *at least* three months after stopping hormonal methods. The following variations are common:

- Longer cycles (usually due to delayed or absent ovulation)
- Short or average length cycles
- Regular or irregular cycles (with more than seven days' variation)

Variations in temperature rise

The progestogen in hormonal contraception slightly increases the resting temperature, so, after stopping your hormonal method, it may take a while for temperatures to settle. Expect some disruption to your temperatures – the following scenarios are all possible (in random sequence):

- There may be normal biphasic cycles with normal-length luteal phases.
- The temperature rise may be delayed.
- There may be fewer than ten raised temperatures (short luteal phase).
- There may be no rise in temperature (monophasic chart).

Extended coverline

In view of the likelihood of erratic temperatures, it is safest to use the extended coverline technique to identify the rise in temperature. Extend the coverline back as far as possible (excluding the first four days of the period). This helps to avoid errors by ensuring that there are more than six low temperatures (see Figure 5.2).

Disturbances to cervical secretions

It can take up to six cycles (or longer) for cervical secretions to return to a normal pattern after stopping any hormonal method. Any of the following scenarios are possible:

- Persistent dry days
- Continuous scant sticky secretions
- Continuous watery or milky secretions
- Intermittent patches of secretions of varying types
- Heavier flow of secretions
- Absence of wetter, transparent, stretchy secretions
- The build-up to peak day may be interrupted
- Peak day may be delayed
- There may be more than one peak day (double or multiple peak)
- Peak day may not be in relation to the temperature rise.

Major cycle disturbances

Major cycle disturbances include cycle lengths of more than 35 days, luteal phases of fewer than ten raised temperatures, and monophasic cycles. Some women's cycles show major disturbances for up to six months (or longer in extreme cases). Cycles are only considered to be back to normal (regular ovulatory pattern) when you have had three *consecutive* biphasic cycles with a luteal phase of ten days or more.

Guidelines to avoid pregnancy after hormonal methods

These guidelines are for use after stopping any form of hormonal contraception, remembering that the late infertile time is always the most effective to avoid pregnancy.

First cycle

No unprotected intercourse even if the chart appears to show a normal biphasic pattern (see Figure 5.1).

Second cycle

- Avoid intercourse during the early infertile time.
- Use the extended coverline to identify the temperature rise (see Figure 5.2 on page 87).
- Intercourse can be resumed after the *fourth* high temperature provided they are **all at least 0.2 °C above the low-phase temperatures** – there must be at least six low temperatures. All high temperatures must be after peak day (see Figure 5.2).

Third and subsequent cycles

- The late infertile time starts on the evening of the *third* high temperature provided it is at least 0.2 °C above the low temperatures. All high temperatures must be after peak day.
- Restrict intercourse to the late infertile time until a regular ovulatory pattern has been re-established.
- When you have had three consecutive biphasic cycles with a luteal phase of ten days or more, you can resume intercourse in the early infertile time using the guidelines for normal fertility found in Chapter 4.

Calculations to identify the start of the fertile time

Start keeping records of cycle length as soon as you stop hormonal methods. You can then use a calculation to identify the start of the fertile time (see Figure 4.1). From your *fourth* cycle onwards, it is safe to have intercourse **up to cycle day 5** provided the first three cycles are 26 days or longer and the period is a true period.

Example charts

The three example charts were recorded by a 29-year-old woman who had come off the combined pill. Figure 5.1 shows her first cycle off the pill – her first bleed (days 1–4) is a hormone withdrawal bleed. This is a 32-day cycle. She has a continuous pattern of milky-white secretions. There is a temperature rise on day 25. She has fewer than ten raised temperatures so this is a short luteal phase. There should be no unprotected intercourse.

Figure 5.2 shows her second post-pill cycle – a 25-day cycle. The temperature rise is on day 14. She has used the extended coverline counting four high temperatures, all of which are 0.2 °C above the low-phase temperatures. Her secretions are a bit erratic, but she notices two days of wetter secretions with peak on day 12. All high temperatures occur after peak day. She could therefore have unprotected intercourse from day 17 until the end of her cycle. The luteal phase is a normal length. From her third cycle onwards, she can have intercourse in the late infertile time after three high temperatures past peak.

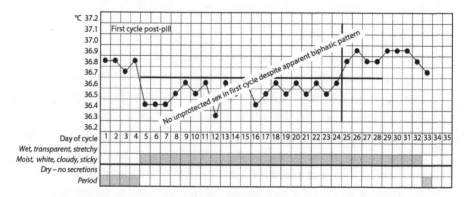

Figure 5.1 First cycle after stopping the combined pill

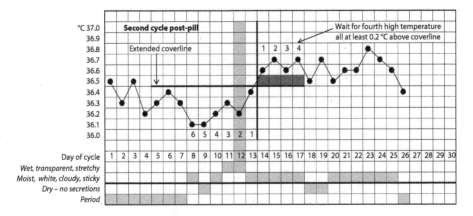

Figure 5.2 Second cycle after stopping the combined pill

Figure 5.3 shows her seventh cycle post-pill – it is 54 days long. Fertility charts span only 40 days, so two charts have been joined together with recordings continuing from one chart to the next. The coverline has been extended right back to day 5. The temperature finally rises on day 42, but at that time she is aware of wet, transparent secretions – her peak day is on day 43. By day 46, there are three high temperatures – they are all at least 0.2 °C above the low-phase readings and they are all after peak day. The late infertile time starts on the evening of day 46. This is a classic example of the importance of waiting for the temperature rise. If this woman was not charting her cycles (and was having unprotected sex), she might assume that she was pregnant based purely on her very long cycle. It is clear from her temperature that ovulation was delayed so delaying her next period. **Never tire of waiting for the temperature rise. The key thing about charting after hormonal methods is to expect the unexpected.**

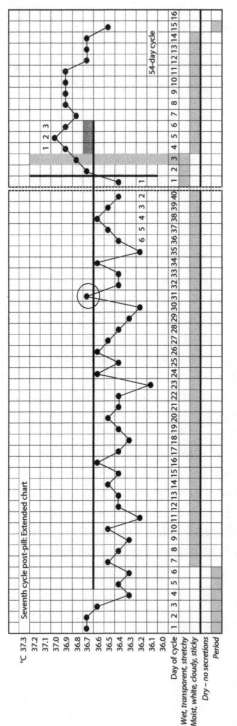

Figure 5.3 Long cycle after stopping the combined pill: the chart has been extended

6

Using fertility awareness methods after childbirth and during breastfeeding

Breast or bottle? How it affects fertility

The choice about whether or not to breastfeed is a personal one – no woman should ever feel pressured into breastfeeding. A mother who bottle-feeds can still have a strong bond with her baby, and modern formula milk is very close nutritionally to breast milk. Ideally all babies would be exclusively breastfed for the first six months, by which time they are ready to start weaning, but shorter durations of breastfeeding are still beneficial. Help and support with breastfeeding is available through NHS maternity services and privately through groups such as the National Childbirth Trust (see Resources). Whether you breastfeed, bottle-feed or combine the two will affect how quickly your fertility returns.

Breastfeeding acts as a natural contraceptive. Women who fully breastfeed may have many months, possibly a year or more without periods. Women who do not breastfeed (or only breastfeed for a short time) may have periods back by about six weeks postnatally, which means ovulation can occur from as early as four weeks after childbirth. While it may be the last thing on your mind when pregnant, it is important to think about what contraception you would like to use after birth so you have an effective family planning method as soon as you start having sex again. Some women feel ready to have intercourse again; others do not want to have intercourse so quickly – it largely depends on your birth experience and how you feel. The six-week postnatal check is an ideal time to discuss issues related to contraception or concerns about sex.

It is best to aim for a gap of about two years between children to give your body time to recover from pregnancy and birth – this is particularly important if you had your baby by caesarean section (C-section). Older women may need to weigh up the health benefits of delaying their next pregnancy against the concerns about declining fertility – this is something to discuss with your doctor.

Lactational amenorrhoea method (LAM)

In the first six months after childbirth, breastfeeding mothers can use the lactational amenorrhoea method (lactation = breastfeeding; amenorrhoea = no periods). Each time a woman suckles her baby, it boosts her prolactin (breastfeeding hormone) level. Prolactin acts on the pituitary gland, switching off the FSH and LH, thus keeping estrogen levels low and preventing ovulation. Prolactin levels fall again after three to four hours, but if the baby suckles frequently, the high level of prolactin is sustained and fertility is suppressed.

LAM is more than 98 per cent effective for the first six months provided that:

- your periods have not returned (you are amenorrhoeic); *and*
- you are fully breastfeeding on demand (day and night); *and*
- your baby is less than six months old.

Once any of these things change, you need to start using another family planning method. This means that you need to think about which method you want to move to before things change so you are ready to switch immediately.

Figure 6.1 shows LAM as a flowchart. Provided you can answer 'yes' to the three key questions, you have less than a 2 per cent chance of pregnancy. LAM applies only in the first six months, so, even if your periods have still not returned by six months, you need to switch to another method. Your doctor or sexual health nurse or clinic will be able to discuss suitable methods which do not interfere with breastfeeding so that you can continue to breastfeed for as long as is right for you and your baby.

The time taken for fertility to return varies from woman to woman and from one breastfeeding experience to another for the same woman – some become fertile again as soon as they start weaning (or before) while others do not regain fertility until the baby is fully weaned. One reason why LAM is so effective is that, during the first six months, most women who are fully breastfeeding will get some bleeding before

Ask yourself these three questions:

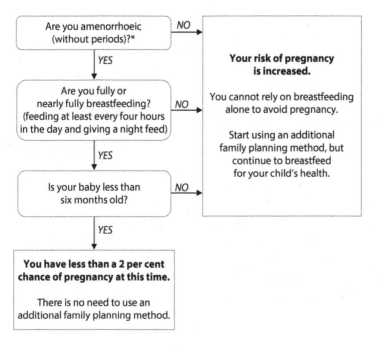

Are you amenorrhoeic (without periods)?* — NO →

Your risk of pregnancy is increased.

You cannot rely on breastfeeding alone to avoid pregnancy.

Start using an additional family planning method, but continue to breastfeed for your child's health.

↓ YES

Are you fully or nearly fully breastfeeding? (feeding at least every four hours in the day and giving a night feed) — NO →

↓ YES

Is your baby less than six months old? — NO →

↓ YES

You have less than a 2 per cent chance of pregnancy at this time.

There is no need to use an additional family planning method.

Note:
* Discount the bleeding after childbirth – this means no bleeding after the first eight weeks.

Figure 6.1 Breastfeeding as a contraceptive method

they ovulate – so a 'period' is your 'wake-up call' for the first sign of fertility. From six months onwards, the majority of women will ovulate before they get their first period – this means that you could go straight from one pregnancy into another without having a period.

How often do I need to breastfeed for LAM to be effective?

You need to breastfeed your baby at least every four hours during the day and at least once during the night (there should not be a gap of more than six hours at night). Most babies will demand this level of feeding anyway, so, provided you are feeding whenever your baby is hungry (or needs comfort), your fertility will naturally be suppressed. Breastfeeding at night releases more prolactin, so when the night feed is dropped, fertility is more likely to return. It is not possible to suppress fertility indefinitely through breastfeeding: even if you continue to breastfeed fully after six months, eventually your fertility will return as your body adjusts.

Can I give my baby a dummy/comforter?

No. Babies breastfeed when they are hungry and also when they need comfort. If you are using LAM, it is important to breastfeed on demand. Do not be tempted to give your baby a dummy as a comforter, because this will reduce suckling time at the breast and could precipitate the return of your fertility.

What happens if I need to express milk?

Expressing milk does not have the same stimulatory effect as a suckling baby, so, if you express milk so that you can be apart from your baby, LAM will not be as effective. Some of the newer electric double pumps (where you express both breasts simultaneously) produce a good yield of milk, but it is not known how much they reduce the effectiveness of LAM.

How do I know when my periods return?

After giving birth (whether vaginally or by caesarean) you will have a bloodstained vaginal discharge for a number of weeks – most of the bleeding comes from the area where the placenta was attached. Bleeding during the first eight weeks (56 days) is not a period – it is known as lochia. It is usually bright red for about five days, then becoming reddish/pinkish brown until about day 12 then yellowish/white until about six weeks after the birth. **Any bleeding after eight weeks, which seems like a period or requires sanitary protection, counts as a period.**

⚠ Abnormal postnatal bleeding

Any loss which is very heavy or has an offensive odour could indicate infection or postnatal complications. Seek urgent medical advice.

Do I need to observe my fertility indicators while using LAM?

No – the beauty of LAM is that no charting is required – any breastfeeding mother can use LAM. You simply need to make sure you can answer 'yes' to those three questions: you have no periods, are fully breastfeeding, and the baby is less than six months old. You can then move from LAM to whatever method you choose. If you want to switch to FAMs, you need to start observing fertility indicators (again) from two weeks before the LAM criteria no longer apply.

Moving from LAM to FAMs

Aim to start charting as soon as you get a period, about two weeks before you start weaning or at five and a half months – whichever comes *earlier*. Help from a fertility awareness practitioner is essential whether you are a new or experienced user. Depending on your breastfeeding pattern and other factors, it could be weeks or months before your normal fertile cycles return.

Each time you breastfeed, it boosts your prolactin which suppresses the ovaries and keeps estrogen levels low – the cervix remains closed and secretions are suppressed. When you reduce the level of breastfeeding, prolactin levels drop, the ovaries become active, estrogen levels rise, and the cervix and its secretions show fertile characteristics. Estrogen levels may fluctuate resulting in intermittent signs of fertility and possibly a few 'false alarms' before the final build-up to ovulation. This can be frustrating, but every sign of potential fertility must be acted on. To recognize fertility, you first need to recognize the infertile pattern associated with breastfeeding.

Recognizing the Basic Infertile Pattern (BIP)

Cervical secretions: establishing the BIP

To establish your Basic Infertile Pattern (BIP), you need to observe either a continuous pattern of dryness or a constant (unchanging) pattern of secretions – there should be no change for *at least* two weeks. If, after two weeks, the pattern has remained constant (e.g. an unchanging pattern of sticky white secretions), then that is your BIP. Occasional dryness during the BIP is infertile too, but if there is *any* change from the BIP which shows more fertile characteristics (e.g. wetter secretions) then this is fertile:

- BIP dryness: *any secretions* are potentially fertile;
- BIP moistness: *any change from the constant pattern* is potentially fertile.

Re-establishing the BIP

When you first establish your BIP, you need a full *two weeks* to make sure that the pattern is unchanging. Once you have established this, respond to any sign of fertility, but once fertile signs are over, you need only *three days* to make sure that your BIP has re-established.

The BIP rule only applies for breastfeeding mothers prior to their first temperature rise. For women of normal fertility *any* secretions are potentially fertile.

Temperature

While breastfeeding, your temperature may show a greater day-to-day variation than during normal fertility (see Figure 6.2). This 'swinging' temperature is characteristic of the infertility associated with breastfeeding. As time progresses (and breastfeeding is reduced), the temperature usually settles to a more stable pattern (sometimes to quite a low level) for a week or two before the temperature rise (Figure 6.3). The swinging temperature is a reassuring sign, but not all women will get this so it cannot be relied on.

Changes in the cervix

It takes up to 12 weeks for the cervix to return to its normal state after childbirth, so start recording cervical changes from 12 weeks onwards. If this is your first birth, then your cervix will feel different compared with the time before pregnancy (see Chapter 3), but you should still be able to distinguish changes. The cervix often provides the earliest sign of approaching fertility:

- Low, firm, closed, tilted cervix: signs of infertility
- First sign of change indicates fertility.

Recognizing signs of fertility

Once you have established your BIP, any change in the cervix or secretions indicates potential fertility:

- Fertility starts at the *first* sign of change – whether from the cervix or secretions.
- Look out for a swinging temperature stabilizing (although this may not occur).

Assume fertility for the duration of the fertile signs and the following *three* days after the BIP has re-established.

Recording on the breastfeeding chart

You can record your fertility indicators on a normal fertility chart (and join charts together), but ideally you would use the longer eight-week breastfeeding chart as shown in Figures 6.2 and 6.3, as it is easier to see a pattern emerging. These are available from most practitioners.

The breastfeeding chart includes space to record the baby's age, number of breastfeeds, additional liquids or solids, and the longest interval between feeds. Note any time you express milk. You can also record details such as immunizations or illness which might affect the intensity of feeds. Get a rough estimate of the time you spend breastfeeding – both full feeds and short comfort feeds. When you start weaning, you will give less breastfeeds with longer intervals between feeds and you will see signs of returning fertility.

Factors which may precipitate the return of fertility

There are a number of different circumstances which may precipitate the return of fertility:

- When breastfeeding becomes less frequent
- When introducing fruit juice, formula milk or small amounts of solid foods
- When your baby first sleeps through the night
- If you become anxious, stressed or ill
- If your baby becomes ill and doesn't feed well.

Unlike normal fertility where stress tends to delay ovulation, the effect of stress during breastfeeding is to allow an *earlier* ovulation – prolactin levels drop, estrogen levels rise and ovulation occurs. Be especially careful if you or your baby are ill.

As a general rule:

- If you wean abruptly, fertility returns rapidly.
- If you wean slowly (over weeks or months), it takes longer for normal fertility to return.

Guidelines to avoid pregnancy during breastfeeding

Before the first temperature rise

- Establish your BIP (unchanging pattern for two weeks):
  - BIP dryness: *any secretions* are potentially fertile
  - BIP moistness: *any change* from the BIP is potentially fertile.
- Restrict intercourse to the evenings so that you can observe secretions throughout the day.
- Mark the day after intercourse with an 'X' to denote a 'wet' (non-intercourse) day because seminal fluid could mask secretions.
- **You can have intercourse during your BIP on *non-consecutive evenings*.**
- Avoid intercourse for the duration of any fertile signs and for the following *three* days.
- Avoid intercourse on any days of bleeding (including spotting) and for the following three days (bleeding could mask secretions).
- Cervix: any change from the low, firm, closed, tilted cervix is fertile.
- **Avoid intercourse at the first sign of returning fertility (whether shown by secretions, bleeding or cervical changes) while the fertile signs last and for three days after your BIP has returned.**

After the first temperature rise

Use the extended coverline to identify the first temperature rise, to make sure that a swinging temperature has settled. Extend the coverline back as far as possible – there must be at least six low temperatures (see Figure 6.3). It is common to have a short luteal phase after the first temperature rise.

Identifying the first temperature rise after childbirth

- Draw a horizontal line on the line immediately above the highest of the low-phase temperatures and extend the coverline.
- You can resume intercourse on the *evening* of the *fourth* high temperature, provided they are *all at least 0.2 °C* above the low readings, and they are *all after peak day*.

Subsequent cycles

In cycles following your first postnatal temperature rise (indicating the return of ovulation), follow the guidelines for normal fertility again.

Early relatively infertile time (pre-ovulatory)

- BIP rules no longer apply.
- Non-consecutive dry evenings are relatively infertile.

Late infertile time (post-ovulatory)

You can resume intercourse on the evening of the *third* high temperature, provided it is at least 0.2 °C above the low-phase temperatures. If it is not at least 0.2 °C higher, wait for a fourth high temperature above the coverline. All high temperatures must be after peak day.

Calculation

Start tracking cycle length to recalculate the start of the fertile time as a cross-check for secretions and cervix (see Chapter 3). You cannot rely on having the same-length cycles as before pregnancy.

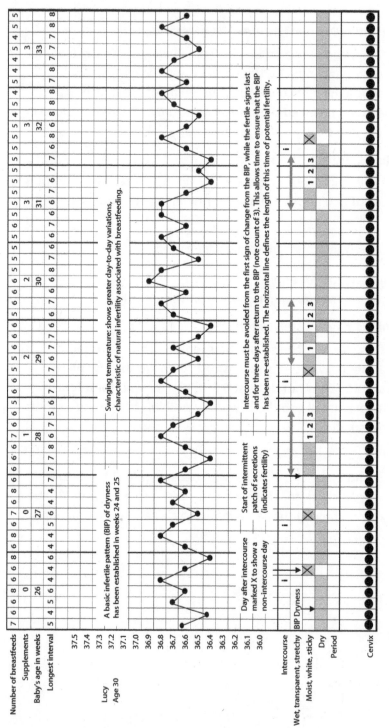

Figure 6.2 Breastfeeding chart showing BIP with intermittent patches of secretions

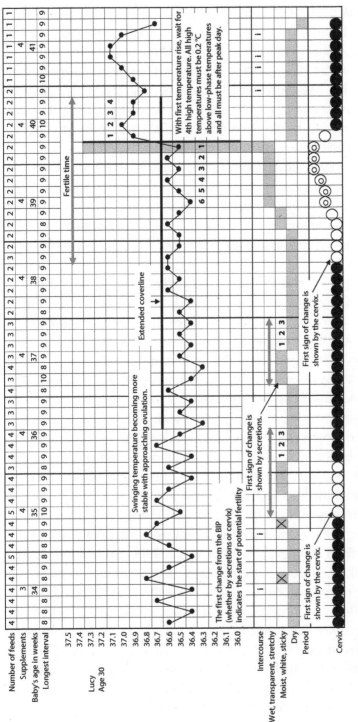

Figure 6.3 Breastfeeding chart showing returning fertility during weaning

The two example charts are from Lucy, a 30-year-old breastfeeding mother who switches from LAM to FAMs at 26 weeks. Figure 6.2 shows her breastfeeding chart from 26 to 33 weeks. Notice that she is still fully breastfeeding at 26 weeks and her periods have not returned. The six-month limit has been reached and she is planning to start weaning soon, so she can no longer rely on LAM. She observed her secretions for two weeks before she started charting (to establish her BIP) and noted that she is consistently dry: her BIP is dryness.

At week 26, Lucy is breastfeeding six to eight times per day with the longest interval between feeds of six hours (at night). She records her BIP of dryness, and her temperature is swinging. She records the evenings she has intercourse and marks the following day with an 'X' (to show a non-intercourse day). Her cervix remains low, firm and closed.

In week 28, Lucy introduces solids – she gradually increases the number of supplements and reduces the number of breastfeeds. She starts to notice intermittent patches of secretions. When she observes any moistness that is not related to intercourse, she avoids intercourse for the duration of change and for the following three days, to make sure that her BIP has re-established. Lucy's temperature continues to show wide day-to-day variations with no sign of a rise. She has indicated the times she is potentially fertile with a horizontal arrow.

Figure 6.3 continues from week 34 to week 41. Lucy is decreasing the number of breastfeeds as she increases solids; her baby is sleeping longer at night, with intervals of up to ten hours. It is a huge bonus to get a good night's sleep, but she is now on high alert for signs of returning fertility. She notices the first cervical change in week 35 – this is the *earliest* sign of change – so she notes this as a sign of potential fertility. By week 38, her cervix is softening, building up to a high, soft, open cervix – this coincides with the build-up of secretions to peak day in week 40. The temperature has stabilized, and it rises to the higher level the day after peak. She counts *four* temperatures at the higher level as this is her first temperature rise after giving birth. All the high temperatures are at least 0.2 °C and they are all after peak day. She has extended her coverline back as far as she can. She is free to have unprotected intercourse day or night from her fourth high temperature after peak day until her next period starts.

FAMs when there is no breastfeeding (or breastfeeding for less than one month)

If a woman does not breastfeed, or breastfeeds for less than one month, her prolactin levels will drop quite rapidly and her ovaries will become active again quickly.

- Most women have their first period about six to eight weeks after delivery (which means that some will ovulate within one month of giving birth).
- The majority of women will ovulate before their first period – it is therefore vital to use an effective contraceptive method from about day 21 after delivery.

Guidelines to avoid pregnancy when not breastfeeding

Start recording your fertility indicators two to three weeks after delivery.

- In the first cycle, you can resume intercourse in the late infertile time from the evening of the *fourth* high temperature, provided *all* high temperatures are at least 0.2 °C above the low-phase temperatures and they are all after peak day.
- In the second and subsequent cycles, you can resume intercourse on the evening of the third high temperature, provided it is at least 0.2 °C above the low-phase temperatures. If it is not at least 0.2 °C higher, wait for a fourth high temperature above the coverline. All high temperatures must be after peak day.
- You can resume intercourse on non-consecutive dry evenings in the early relatively infertile time from the second cycle onwards.
- You will need to start collecting information about cycle lengths again so you can recalculate the start of your fertile time (see Chapter 3).

7

Using fertility awareness methods when approaching the menopause

The terminology around the menopause can be confusing. The word 'menopause' literally means 'end of menstruation' – the final period. In the UK, the average age at menopause is 51. The time leading up to the menopause is known as the perimenopause and is the time when most women in their forties start having irregular cycles and menopausal symptoms. The perimenopause typically lasts about four to five years starting from the first sign of change from normal ovulatory cycles until ovulation and periods stop completely and then for one year after the final period. A woman is said to be *post*-menopausal (past the menopause) when she has had one full year without periods.

The age at menopause tends to run in families, so if you know when your mother went through menopause, this will give you an idea of your own likely menopausal age. Women who smoke go through menopause about two years earlier than non-smokers. If the menopause occurs before the age of 40, this is considered a premature menopause and may require treatment (with hormone replacement therapy known as HRT). Women who have surgery to remove their ovaries experience an immediate menopause and similarly may require HRT to help manage symptoms.

Although natural pregnancy in women over 50 is rare, it is important to use an effective contraceptive method until you are advised by your doctor that it is safe to stop – this is normally two years after menopause if you are under 50 and one year after menopause if you are over 50. All women over 55 can stop contraception. If you have charted your cycles during normal fertility, you should be able to identify early perimenopausal changes, but, even if you are an experienced FAM user, you will need additional help to interpret your charts. It is certainly not an easy time to start using FAMs, but it is possible with a lot of patience and expert help. It is not possible to use

FAMs if you are using any form of HRT. Note that fertility monitors and ovulation predictor kits which measure estrogen and LH in urine are not suitable for perimenopausal women.

Hormonal changes

The menopause occurs when the ovaries stop responding to FSH and LH from the pituitary gland, the follicles stop growing and maturing, and the level of estrogen and progesterone drops – it is the fall in these hormones that causes menopausal symptoms. The ovaries normally shut down gradually. If the ovaries do not respond to a certain level of FSH, then more FSH is produced to 'shout louder' at the ovaries. Sometimes there is a response, follicles grow, estrogen levels rise, and an egg is released, but at other times the ovaries remain stubbornly 'deaf' to the messages, follicles fail to grow and there is no ovulation. Over time the ovaries become increasingly dormant, estrogen levels remain low, there is no ovulation and eventually periods stop completely. A blood test to check your hormone levels can give an idea of how you are progressing through the menopausal stages but cannot give a definitive answer about whether you are permanently infertile.

Perimenopausal symptoms

Common perimenopausal symptoms include hot flushes, night sweats, sleep disturbance, headaches, fatigue, mood swings, anxiety, depression, joint pains, palpitations, dry skin and hair, loss of libido, vaginal dryness, pain during intercourse and urinary frequency. Longer-term health risks of reduced estrogen include osteoporosis (loss of bone density) and an increased risk of heart attacks and strokes. Staying fit and active and maintaining a healthy weight helps most women to get through the menopause with minimal trouble, but if symptoms are disturbing and do not improve over time, then seek medical advice. The first approach may be modifications to diet and lifestyle, but your GP can discuss the pros and cons of HRT. See NHS Website A-Z Women's Health / Menopause (listed in Resources).

Cycle changes: what to expect

The key thing with the perimenopause is to 'expect the unexpected' – this is a time of major hormonal change. Some women continue to have regular ovulatory cycles then periods stop abruptly, but most experience varying degrees of cycle disturbance. Anticipate variations in the length of cycles: some will be ovulatory but others will be anovulatory. Expect changes in the length of pre-ovulation and post-ovulation phases, reduced amounts of secretions and changes in vaginal bleeding. Different cycle types occur randomly in a variable sequence of fertile and infertile cycles.

Variations in cycle length

- Average-length cycles
- Short cycles (23 days or less) – these are often an early sign of perimenopausal changes
- Irregular cycles (more than seven days difference in the length of consecutive cycles)
- Very long cycles (gaps of 60 days or more between 'periods') – these are more common in the later perimenopausal years

Biphasic charts

- Temperature rise can occur early (early ovulation)
- Temperature rise may be delayed (late ovulation)
- Luteal phase may be short (fewer than ten raised temperatures)
- Blood loss is varied but may be heavy and prolonged

Monophasic charts

- No rise in temperature (indicating no ovulation in that cycle)
- Cycles are often longer but they may be average length or short
- Blood loss may be very light but it is sometimes heavier and of longer duration

Effects on cervical secretions

- Decreasing amounts of slippery stretchy secretions
- Increasing number of dry days

- Intermittent patches of sticky white secretions
- Secretions may start very early in the cycle (warning of early ovulation)
- Very short build-up to peak day

Effects on temperature

- Variations in the day of temperature rise – earlier or later than usual
- Short luteal phases
- Monophasic charts

Changes in vaginal bleeding

- Heavy prolonged bleeding with clots
- Sudden brief or more prolonged episodes of bleeding or 'flooding'
- Very light bleeding
- Spotting either between periods or instead of a proper period
- Consider whether this change in bleeding pattern requires medical advice (see caution below).

Is it a true period?

It is only considered a 'true period' if there was a temperature rise 10–16 days earlier. If there was no temperature rise (no ovulation), then after some time your hormone levels will drop anyway and you will get a bleed – this is a hormone withdrawal bleed and *not* a true period.

During the perimenopause consider any bleeding to be potentially fertile. Bleeding could be a sign of estrogen activity and ovulation; or, if it is true period, bleeding could mask the first appearance of secretions in a short cycle.

⚠ Caution

If periods are getting further apart, shorter and lighter, then there is generally no cause for concern. However, if the time between periods is becoming shorter, and the bleeding is longer and heavier or if there is any unusual bleeding or bleeding between periods, or after intercourse, seek medical advice. The most likely explanation is hormonal changes but there are other possible causes including gynaecological cancers. Any woman who has vaginal bleeding more than one year after her final period should seek prompt medical advice.

Recording on the perimenopause chart

The fertility indicators are recorded in the usual way (see the Appendix). Your FAM practitioner may have specialized 16-week charts which make it easier to observe changes over a longer time frame. Menopausal symptoms can be recorded on the chart to help monitor their impact on general wellbeing.

Recognizing signs of infertility

The key to successful use of FAMs when approaching the menopause lies not so much in identifying fertility but in confidently identifying the increasingly lengthy times of infertility.

- **Cervical secretions**: there may be many dry days, often continuing to be persistently dry for a number of weeks.
- **Cervix**: the cervix will remain low, firm, closed and tilted.
- **Temperature**: the temperature remains on one level – a monophasic chart indicating the absence of ovulation.
- **Calculation**: once cycles start to become irregular, then calculations to identify the start of the fertile time will not be accurate, so these can no longer be relied on.

Recognizing signs which may indicate fertility

- **Cervical secretions**: any change from dryness indicates fertility.
- **Period or bleeding**: all bleeding is potentially fertile, because it could either be associated with ovarian activity or, if it is a true period, then the bleeding could mask the start of secretions in a very short cycle

- **Cervix**: the first change from the low, firm, closed, tilted cervix indicates fertility. The earliest sign of fertility may be shown by either the first sign of secretions or the first change in the cervix, whichever comes *earlier*.
- **Temperature**: biphasic temperature with a normal length luteal phase (ten or more high temperatures)

Guidelines to avoid pregnancy during the perimenopause

These guidelines are for use by women whose cycles are showing signs of change from normal ovulatory cycles. They should only be used under close supervision by a FAM practitioner. The emphasis here is on finding the early and late infertile times.

Early relatively infertile time

- Intercourse is permitted in the early dry days on *non-consecutive evenings.*
- *Any* bleeding or spotting:
  - If the bleed is a true period, avoid intercourse for the duration of the period (to ensure that the bleeding is not masking any secretions). Great caution is required here as there can be a rapid build-up of secretions to peak day.
  - If the bleed is not a true period, avoid intercourse for the duration of the bleed and for the following three days to establish a return to dryness. Intercourse can be resumed on the evening of the fourth dry day.
- Avoid intercourse at the first sign of change from dryness or the first change from an infertile cervix, whichever comes *earlier*. Avoid intercourse for the duration of the fertile signs and for *three* days after the return to dryness (and an infertile cervix).

Late infertile time

- Intercourse can be resumed on the evening of the third high temperature provided it is at least 0.2 °C above the low-phase temperatures and all high temperatures are after peak day.

- There must be at least six low temperatures, but try extending the coverline backwards as far as possible, excluding the first four temperatures of the period.
- Once the late infertile time has started, you can have sex day or night until the start of the next period.

Figure 7.1 shows a perimenopausal chart recorded by Zoe, a 46-year-old experienced user. The chart spans eight weeks. Zoe has noted that there was no temperature rise in her previous cycle, so the bleed is not a true period (a possible sign of ovarian activity). There was no intercourse during the bleed and for the following three days (note the count of 1, 2, 3). Intercourse was then permitted on dry days on non-consecutive evenings. She and her partner had intercourse (circled) on day 8, so the following day is marked as moist (possibly seminal fluid – but it could be masking secretions) – she has marked it with an 'X' (non-intercourse day). They continued having intercourse in the evenings only on non-consecutive dry days. On day 15, Zoe noticed secretions that were not related to intercourse – she therefore avoided intercourse that day and for the following three days. The cervix stayed low, firm, closed and tilted until day 23, when it softened – this was the first sign of change so the fertile time had started. The fertile time continued until day 31 when she had three high temperatures – the third temperature was at least 0.2 °C above the low temperatures and all high temperatures were after peak day. Note the short luteal phase. They avoided intercourse during Zoe's period but resumed again on day 6 when she felt confident of dryness and a closed cervix. The following day, her cervix softened, giving the first sign of change. She had a very short build-up of secretions before peak on day 11 and the temperature rise on day 12. The fertile time lasted from day 7 until day 14. They could then have intercourse day or night until Zoe's next period started.

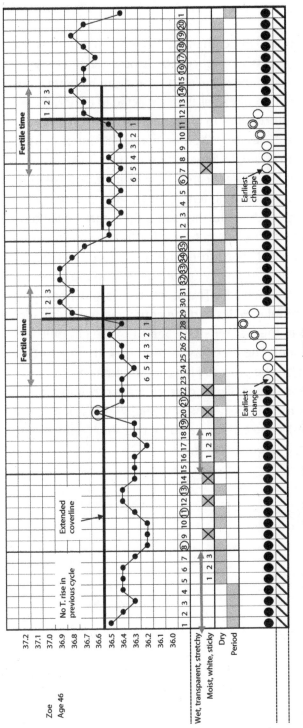

Figure 7.1 Perimenopausal chart recorded by a 46-year-old experienced FAM user

Risks of pregnancy

Fertility is significantly reduced in perimenopausal women, but there will still be many ovulatory cycles where conception is possible and these occur randomly. Intercourse in the early infertile time can be particularly risky because ovulation can occur earlier than expected in a short cycle and there is often only a short build-up of secretions before peak day. In practice, many of these cycles have short or inadequate luteal phases but others will have a normal-length luteal phase so they could sustain a pregnancy. Some couples feel more secure if they limit intercourse to the late infertile time (following three high temperatures after peak day), but as cycles get longer and periods are further apart, there may be limited time for unprotected intercourse, which can be frustrating.

Figure 7.2 shows a series of charts from an experienced FAM user. The top series of charts show Anne's cycles at age 46 and the bottom series show her cycles five years later. The darker blocks show episodes of bleeding. Note the irregular cycles and the combination of biphasic and monophasic cycles in the first series. By age 51, Anne has only one biphasic cycle (in June). She then has six months without a further temperature rise, although she does still have intermittent bleeds and patches of secretions. She is most likely to be permanently infertile now, but she waits to ensure that she has one year after her final bleed (which was in December) – she can now assume that she is permanently infertile and she can finally stop charting.

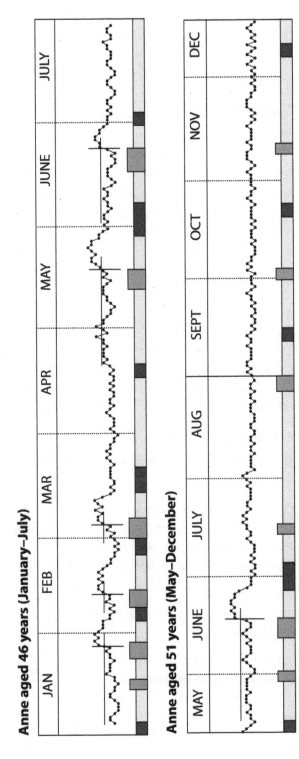

Figure 7.2 Cycles recorded by a 46-year-old woman and the same woman five years later

8

Planning pregnancy and preconception care

Pregnancy is the result of sexual intercourse or by assisted conception at the fertile time. Pregnancy lasts around 280 days or nine months. It is dated from the first day of the last period to the date of delivery. Pregnancy is divided into three trimesters: each roughly three months long.

Thinking about pregnancy and deciding to have a baby

Research and surveys show that while people plan most carefully for clothing, weddings, buying a car and holidays – often in minute detail – most do not 'plan' for pregnancy. It is seen as something that will just happen, even though this is one of the most important life decisions you will ever make.

Some things to think about

When making a decision to have a baby, it may be helpful to consider the following things:

- **Your life now**: What is most important to you in your life at the moment – work, career progression, education, independence, money, friends, pleasure, your partner, your family?
- **Your future**: What are your hopes and aims for the future? Think about all aspects of your life.

How would these things be affected if you became pregnant? Ask yourself the following questions:

- Am I ready to be a parent and bring up a child?
- Do I have a partner who wants to be a parent?
- Do I need a partner to have children?

- If I have a baby, what things might I have to stop doing that I enjoy?
- Can I/we afford to have children?
- What support would I have from family/friends?
- Will I lose my independence?

Are you feeling pressured to have a baby?

- By a partner whose views may be very different to yours?
- By friends, parents or others?
- Because you are concerned about your 'biological clock'?
- By expectations of society – 'because it's what you do'?
- As an insurance policy for growing old?
- Because you do not want to regret not having a child?

Many women worry that, once they have made the decision and start trying for a baby, they will not become pregnant; this is magnified when pregnancy does not happen immediately.

Mostly we spend much more time thinking about how to prevent pregnancy – what contraception to use, which is best, whether it will work and so on – and suddenly these concerns are replaced with concerns about wanting to get pregnant and why it has not happened straight away. Questions immediately arise: 'Am I doing something wrong?' 'Did the abortion I had make me infertile?' 'How can I be sure my tubes were not blocked by that infection?' 'Am I too old?' 'Is there something wrong with my partner's sperm?' 'Are we having enough sex? 'Does it matter if the seminal fluid comes out after sex?' Such thoughts and worries are common. What is important to know is that most women will become pregnant, but it can take time and this is normal.

Fast facts

For every 100 couples trying for a baby:

- Around 30 will conceive in the first month.
- Around 75 will conceive within six months.
- Around 80–90 will conceive within one year. The remaining 10–20 will take longer, or may require help to get pregnant.

This is the time to relax and enjoy your decision to try for a baby – to enjoy good sex and lovemaking without any pressures. However, don't turn it into 'Project Baby' to the exclusion of everything else. Use this time to think about how you might enjoy your new role as a mother or father and how a new baby or another baby will fit into your life. Consider what you may have to change to ensure a happy and healthy pregnancy. This may include diet and lifestyle changes and how best to manage any stress you might be feeling.

How will I know I am pregnant? The pregnancy test

The earliest and most reliable sign of pregnancy for women with a regular menstrual cycle is a missed period. Sometimes women who are pregnant still have a 'period', but it will be shorter or lighter than normal. A pregnancy test will confirm a pregnancy. This test looks for the hormone human chorionic gonadotrophin (hCG), which is released once the embryo has implanted into the endometrium.

You can carry out a pregnancy test from the first day of a missed period. Tests carried out earlier than this are not always accurate. Sometimes the test does not show positive until a period is at least a week late. If you don't have regular periods, the earliest time you can do a test is 21 days from the last time you had unprotected sex.

Pregnancy tests are usually very accurate; a positive test is almost always correct. A woman can sometimes get a negative result if the test is carried out too early or not correctly, even though she may be pregnant. Pregnancy tests that you can buy are just as effective as the tests carried out by your GP, practice nurse or hospital.

It's all in the genes – where do we come from?

The genes we inherit from our biological parents impact on how we look, what our characters are like and our physical and mental abilities. Genes are contained in chromosomes – tiny thread-like structures found in every living cell in the body. We normally inherit 23 chromosomes from each parent, giving a total of 46 – arranged as 23 pairs. Every cell in the human body contains 46 chromosomes except for a woman's eggs and a man's sperm. An egg and a sperm each contain 22 chromosomes and one sex chromosome. The egg's sex chromosome is known as the X chromosome and the sperm's sex chromosome can be either an X or a Y chromosome. It is the sperm's sex chromosome that determines the biological sex of a baby. A simple way to look at it is like this:

- If the egg is fertilized by a sperm containing an X sex chromosome, the baby will be a female.

  Mother X + Father X = XX = Female

- If the sperm contains a Y sex chromosome the baby will be a male.

  Mother X + Father Y = XY = Male

Can you influence the sex of your baby?

Many people ask if there is anything you can do to choose or influence the sex of a baby. There have been many popular theories regarding sex selection based around the fact that sperm bearing the Y sex chromosome (male) are lighter and smaller and swim faster, compared with those bearing the X sex chromosome (female). There is no reliable scientific evidence to support claims made for choosing the sex of your baby naturally, such as when you have sex, sexual positions or diet.

If there is a medical or genetic reason why you should avoid having a child of a particular sex, then specialized sex selection techniques are available as part of assisted conception such as in-vitro fertilization (IVF). It is not legal in the UK to use these techniques to have a child of the desired sex for social reasons or family balancing.

Preparing for conception and pregnancy

Your health and the health of your future child

Your chances of becoming pregnant and having a full-term pregnancy and a good-sized healthy baby are better if you and your partner are as fit and healthy as possible. Preparation for pregnancy is important. To optimize your chances of a healthy pregnancy, ideally give yourselves about three months to prepare for pregnancy before attempting to conceive. This timing gives you the opportunity to consider your health and to address any lifestyle issues. What you eat, being a healthy weight, how much you exercise, and whether you or your partner smoke or drink alcohol are all-important factors to think about once you have decided to try for a baby. The NHS website Health A–Z and Tommy's Planning for Pregnancy tool have good information to support you at this time (see Resources).

Your preconception consultation with your GP

Many women do not think about seeing their GP when thinking about having a baby. It is, however, a good idea to see your GP or practice nurse. This gives you an opportunity to discuss any specific health issues and concerns you may have about your fertility, conception, pregnancy or childbirth. It also gives you an opportunity to consider the impact of pregnancy and raising a child on your relationship and lifestyle.

Some of the aspects, which may be discussed, include:

- Rubella – you can ask if you are unsure about whether you were previously vaccinated against MMR (combined measles, mumps and rubella)
- Other vaccinations such as flu, Coronavirus and travel
- Folic acid – a supplement recommended in early pregnancy and when trying for a baby
- Vitamin D – you may need supplements if you are at risk of low Vitamin D levels
- Sexual health check – an opportunity to consider any symptoms or risk factors; checks may include screening for chlamydia, gonorrhoea and syphilis, hepatitis B or C, and HIV
- Cervical screening – you may need a test if it is due or overdue
- Medical conditions – consider any impact on your health or the health of a future baby
- Concerns about a partner's medical conditions or issues and need for consultation
- Psychological and mental health – consider any history of severe anxiety, depression or concerns about postnatal depression
- Any disabilities and specialist help that may be required
- Prescribed medication – this may need to be modified
- Non-prescribed medicines

- Past surgery – to reassure you or discuss further investigations
- Gynaecological conditions or symptoms requiring investigation
- Menstrual cycle history and concerns about irregularities
- Stopping contraception or change from a long-acting contraceptive method to a short-acting method
- Lifestyle advice: smoking, alcohol, caffeine, recreational drugs, weight, exercise, work and travel
- Managing stress
- Sexual and relationship difficulties and referral for help
- Your understanding of the fertility cycle and frequency of sex
- How long to try for a baby before seeking investigations.

Physical, emotional or sexual abuse

Your consultation with your GP also gives you an opportunity to talk about any concerns about domestic violence or physical, sexual, psychological or emotional abuse. Many women feel reluctant to talk about this, but it is important to do so, as very often abuse increases when pregnant. Your doctor can offer support and refer you for specialist help or you can call the National Domestic Abuse (freephone) Helpline (Refuge). In addition, a code word scheme – Ask for ANI (Action Needed Immediately) has been set up by the UK government to provide a discreet way for people suffering with domestic abuse to signal they need emergency help from the safety of their local pharmacy.

For all up-to-date information and advice about health when planning a pregnancy or when pregnant go to the pregnancy section on the NHS website Health A–Z (see Resources).

Vaccinations – what do I need to know?

Rubella immunity

The rubella (German measles) virus can seriously damage a baby's heart, eyes and ears if contracted during pregnancy, particularly during the first 12 weeks. You will probably be immune (protected against the infection) for life if you had rubella as a child or had a rubella vaccination at school. Most babies are now given the MMR vaccine (combined measles, mumps and rubella), owing to the damage these three infections can cause to adults and pregnant women.

In view of the very serious nature of rubella in pregnancy, it is very important to check that you are immune before you become pregnant. If you are not sure, ask your doctor about this and they can do a blood test to check your level of antibodies to rubella. If you are not immune, your doctor or nurse will give you the MMR vaccine. You should have this injection at least one month before you start trying to conceive. You cannot have this vaccination once you are pregnant.

Flu vaccination

It is recommended that all pregnant women should have the flu vaccine whatever stage of pregnancy they are at. There is good evidence that pregnant women have a higher chance of pregnancy complications if they get flu, particularly in the later stages of pregnancy. Research also shows that having the flu vaccine while pregnant passes some protection to the baby which lasts for the first few months of their lives.

Coronavirus Disease vaccination

COVID-19 is a virus that emerged worldwide in 2019. It is a highly contagious respiratory disease caused by SARS-CoV-2. SARS stands for Severe Acute Respiratory Syndrome. Over time, viruses mutate and change and there are now different variants of SARS-CoV-2. The information in this book refers to COVID-19. All women and men are recommended to have COVID-19 vaccinations and boosters when necessary. Vaccination is safe for women planning pregnancy and for women who are pregnant. Pregnant women are more at risk of becoming seriously ill from COVID-19 if they do not have the vaccination. Importantly, the COVID-19 vaccination has no known effect on women's or men's fertility or ability to have children. For full information, see sections on coronavirus on the NHS and RCOG websites (see Resources).

Research suggests that some women undergo changes to their menstrual cycles after having the COVID-19 vaccine or COVID infection. These changes are temporary, and periods return to normal after one or two cycles. It is not known if these changes relate to COVID or to the fact that this reflects normal variation in bleeding patterns that occur but are not often discussed. Women who are charting their fertility sometimes notice a spike in temperature the day after a COVID vaccination.

It is likely that there will be new contagious diseases in the future. Considerable worldwide research is ongoing to address how such infections, diseases and pandemics will be managed.

Travel vaccinations and Zika virus

For information on travel vaccinations including the Zika virus see Travel section on page 145.

Folic acid supplements

Folate or synthetic folic acid is a member of the vitamin B family and is important for a baby's development in the early weeks of pregnancy. Many foods naturally contain folate such as leafy green vegetables and fruits such as oranges. Some foods are also fortified or enriched with folate such as some breads, juices and cereals. These are important to eat when planning pregnancy and during pregnancy. However, it is difficult to get the amount of folate recommended for a healthy pregnancy from food alone, which is why medical advice for all women planning pregnancy is to take additional folic acid in for the form of a daily supplement. You should take 0.4 mg (400 mcg) of folic acid from the time you stop contraception to the twelfth week of pregnancy.

Folic acid helps prevent serious abnormalities of the brain and spine. It also has a protective effect against other congenital defects including cleft lip and palate and, if taken for a year, may protect against preterm delivery. You can buy folic acid from your pharmacy or you may be given it on prescription from your doctor. Many pregnancy and preconception multivitamins contain folic acid but check they contain 400 mcg of folic acid.

If you have had a previous pregnancy affected by a neural tube defect such as spina bifida, or you or your partner or a close relative has a neural tube defect, or you have epilepsy or diabetes, you should take a higher dose of folic acid. Women with a twin pregnancy and women who have a body mass index (BMI) over 30 also require a higher dose of folic acid. Some women with chronic health conditions which affect absorption, such as coeliac disease, diabetes mellitus, sickle cell anaemia, thalassaemia, and liver or kidney disease, may also need a higher dose of folic acid and may have to take it for a longer time. Women taking an anti-retroviral medicine for HIV may also need a higher dose of folic acid. Your doctor or practice nurse will advise you.

Vitamin D

Our main source of vitamin D is through the action of sunlight on bare skin. All adults, including pregnant and breastfeeding women, need 10 mcg of vitamin D each day. Vitamin D is important to regulate the amount of calcium and phosphate which are needed for strong bones and good skin. There is a link between vitamin D deficiency and problems with ovulation, polycystic ovarian syndrome (PCOS), and miscarriage.

Women who have limited exposure to sunlight, such as women who are housebound or who usually remain covered when outdoors, are advised to take a supplement of vitamin D in pregnancy. Sometimes it is advised to take vitamin D during the winter months as there is less sunlight at this time. Women of South Asian, African, African Caribbean or Middle Eastern family origin are less efficient at making vitamin D in the UK climate because melanin (the substance responsible for skin colour which protects the skin against harmful sun damage) slows the production of vitamin D. Women who have a BMI over 30 are also advised to take extra vitamin D. Aim to get out in the sun for at least 20 minutes a day without sunscreen to boost your vitamin D; however, if you are very fair-skinned, do take care, as excessive sun exposure can be damaging. Ask your doctor about a blood test to check your vitamin D level and whether you need any supplementation. Vitamin D is fat-soluble and is harmful if supplements are taken in excess. You may be advised to have a repeat blood test to keep an eye on your levels.

Minerals: iodine, selenium and iron

Iodine is a trace element found in sea water, rocks and some types of soil. It helps to make the thyroid hormones which keep the metabolic rate healthy. Iodine is important in the early weeks of pregnancy for the development of the baby's brain. Low iodine levels during pregnancy can affect a child's IQ. Good food sources include sea fish, shellfish (raw shellfish should be avoided once pregnant), dairy products and iodized salt. Iodine is also found in cereals and grains but the amount varies depending on the amount of iodine in the soil. Other minerals such as selenium help with the normal functioning of the thyroid gland, which is essential for fertility and prevention of miscarriage. Selenium is found in Brazil nuts, seafood, eggs, garlic, onions, broccoli, mushrooms and asparagus. Iron is important as low levels cause anaemia, which results in tiredness, lack of energy and stress. Ensure your diet is rich in iron-containing foods such as lean meat, green leafy vegetables, dried fruits and nuts. Many breakfast cereals contain added iron.

If you are living with a medical condition, it is important to be aware of any foods (or supplements) to avoid. For example, if you have thyroid disease you should not take iodine; or if you have haemachromatosis (an inherited condition where iron levels build up in the body), you should not take iron. Always check with your doctor, nurse or pharmacist.

Multi-vitamin supplement

If you are eating a healthy balanced diet with lots of fresh fruit and vegetables, then supplementation should not be necessary; however, some women (and men) like to take a good-quality multi-vitamin and mineral supplement as part of their daily diet. Standard multi-vitamins may contain too much retinol (the animal form of vitamin A), which can increase the risk of birth defects, particularly heart, brain and face defects, so make sure you take a supplement which is suitable for pregnancy. Ask your doctor or pharmacist for a recommendation. This may contain beta-carotene, which is the safe vegetable form of vitamin A. Some vitamin A is important for the fetal brain and eye health and development. Good dietary sources are eggs (well cooked) and butter, as well as carotene-rich foods.

All preconception and pregnancy multivitamins should contain the recommended dose of 400 mcg folic acid (always check). If you are taking a preconception multi-vitamin containing folic acid, you do not need to take additional folic acid tablets. Vitamin supplements are no substitute for a good diet including fresh fruit and vegetables, but it is very difficult to obtain the recommended 400 mcg of folic acid from diet alone so this must be supplemented.

Some vitamins (A, D, E and K) are soluble in fat and so can accumulate in your body to dangerous levels if you take too much, whereas the B group of vitamins and vitamin C (ascorbic acid) are water soluble so tend to get flushed through your body. Vitamin C helps to protect egg and sperm cells, but high doses (over 1,000 mg per day) of vitamin C are not recommended and may reduce cervical secretions. It is important to keep to recommended limits when taking vitamins and mineral supplements.

Vegetarian, vegan or special diets in pregnancy

Whatever food preferences we have, as long as you have a balanced and mixed vegetarian diet you should have enough nutrients for you and your baby. If you have a vegan diet or a restricted diet (e.g. if you have gluten intolerance), you should just check your dietary needs with your doctor or practice nurse.

Sexual health checks

If you or your partner have ever been at risk of a sexually transmitted infection (STI), or think you might have an STI, or you are just not sure and want to find out, you can get confidential advice and help from a genitourinary medicine clinic (GUM), a sexual health clinic or your general practice. Some STIs (such as chlamydia and gonorrhoea) can affect your chances of getting pregnant, and if not treated they can be passed on to your baby during pregnancy or birth. Some infections are 'silent', meaning they do not have obvious symptoms so can go unnoticed. STIs are easy to detect and if treated early will not affect your chances of getting pregnant.

Bacterial STIs such as chlamydia and gonorrhoea, if left untreated or treated late after getting the infection, can cause pelvic inflammatory disease (PID). This is when the infection causes damage to the reproductive organs. If you have been treated for PID and are having difficulty in conceiving, you may need to see a fertility specialist to check the health of your reproductive organs. The delicate fallopian tubes can easily be damaged or blocked by infection.

Cystitis

If you suffer from recurrent cystitis (inflammation of the bladder or urine infection) or symptoms of vaginal 'thrush' (yeast infection), see your doctor to get an accurate diagnosis and make sure you and your partner are treated.

Typical symptoms of cystitis include pain when you pass urine and passing urine frequently. You may also have lower abdominal pain, blood in your urine and a fever (high temperature). Your urine may also become cloudy or smell offensive. Bacteria from your bowel cause most urine infections. Mild cases of cystitis may resolve spontaneously (with painkillers and plenty of fluids) but antibiotic treatment may be needed.

Cystitis is relatively common in women but much less so in men due to the anatomical difference in the length of the urethra. Men who suffer from urological symptoms including passing urine more frequently, or aches in the testicles should see their doctor. Prostatitis (inflammation of the prostate gland) is common in men. As the prostate gland contributes to the seminal fluid, this can affect fertility and should always be investigated.

Thrush

Candida albicans, a yeast, can cause thrush which develops in the vagina and on the male and female genitals. It is not sexually transmitted but can sometimes develop after sex. It is a very common cause of abnormal vaginal discharge. This yeast lives harmlessly on the skin and in the mouth, gut and vagina. Normally it is kept under control, but occasionally conditions change and signs and symptoms of thrush develop. This is particularly so during pregnancy and after using antibiotics (such as for cystitis). Three out of four women will have thrush some time in their lives, but it is much less common in men.

Many women buy treatments for thrush if they notice an unusual vaginal discharge, but only about one-third of the women who think they have thrush are correct in their self-diagnosis. Other infections such as bacterial vaginosis (BV) are very common. It is important to get a check from your GP, practice nurse or from a sexual health clinic, especially if the symptoms do not go away.

Bacterial vaginosis (BV)

BV is a bacterial infection that only affects women. Women with BV tend to have less of the normal vaginal bacteria (lactobacilli); an overgrowth of other types of bacteria, and a change in the vaginal pH (acid/alkaline balance) making it more alkaline. You might notice a change in your usual vaginal secretions. This may increase, become thin and watery or change to a white/grey colour and develop a strong, unpleasant, fishy smell, especially after intercourse. BV is not usually associated with soreness, itching or irritation. Around half of women with BV will not have any signs or symptoms, or may not be aware of them.

BV is diagnosed by examination and a swab test. Treatment may be antibiotics or a vaginal cream or gel. For many women BV will go away by itself. However, if you are planning pregnancy, it is important to get it treated. Although there is no evidence that BV affects your chances of conception, the untreated infection may cause miscarriage, preterm birth or a low birth-weight baby. One in three women will get BV at some point in their life. It is not an STI but can develop after you have had sex. Using scented soaps, bubble bath, vaginal deodorant or antiseptics can alter the normal pH in your vagina, which may then increase your risk of BV.

Cervical screening

The NHS in the UK provides cervical screening for all women from the age of 25 or 20 – the starting age varies in the four nations. Screening is carried out every three to five years. The test involves checking your cervix for any early changes which, if left untreated, could lead to cervical cancer. You may be offered a cervical screening (which used to be called a smear test) if you have not had one in the last three years. If any changes are found, it is easier to treat abnormal cells when you are not pregnant. Check if you are up to date with your cervical screening, and if not, ask for a test before you start trying for a baby. Your general practice can arrange this. If you have any unusual bleeding such as bleeding between periods or bleeding after sex (post-coital bleeding) always get this checked by your doctor. For more information see the Cancer screening website or the NHS website Health A–Z. Vaccination for HPV (human papillomavirus) is now routinely offered to young girls and boys. HPV is the name of a common group of viruses, and there are many types. The vaccination protects against the HPV that causes genital warts, and it has been shown to reduce the incidence of cervical cancer and some other reproductive cancers such as cancer of the vulva, vagina and penis.

Medical conditions

Talk to your doctor about how your pregnancy might be affected if:

- You have any medical condition such as diabetes, epilepsy, thyroid problems, renal disease, bowel disease or any allergies such as asthma or eczema
- You have any mental health conditions, for example bipolar disorder. Talk to your doctor or your psychiatric specialist. Some areas have specialist perinatal mental health teams and support. See also information from the pregnancy charity – Tommy's Pregnancy and Post-birth Wellbeing Plan (see Resources). This plan helps you start thinking about how you feel emotionally and what support you might need in your pregnancy and after birth. Tommy's specializes in promoting healthy pregnancy and researching the causes and prevention of miscarriage.
- You are taking any prescribed medication, as this may need to be altered. Your doctor will discuss the benefits and risks of drugs such as antidepressants when trying to conceive. Never stop prescribed medication without first consulting your doctor.
- You have a history of heart or circulatory problems, such as high blood pressure (hypertension) or thrombosis (blood clots).
- You or your partner has any hereditary conditions in the family such as sickle cell anaemia, sickle cell trait, thalassaemia, cystic fibrosis or muscular dystrophy.
- You have any known gynaecological problems, such as endometriosis, polycystic ovarian syndrome (PCOS) or fibroids.
- You have had any problems in previous pregnancies including miscarriage, infections or a baby of low birth weight or born prematurely.
- Your doctor can also talk to you about genetic counselling if you or your partner has an inherited condition.

If you are under the care of a specialist doctor for a medical condition, then it is really important to talk to them before you try for a baby. Your specialist may want to liaise with your general practitioner and obstetrician to ensure your medical condition is well controlled and to optimize your health and the health of your baby.

Medicines and drugs

If you take medicines for any reason, tell your doctor or pharmacist that you are planning to get pregnant as some drugs may affect the developing baby. This includes using prescribed medicines or over-the-counter medicines for acne or weight loss. If you are taking medication for epilepsy or a mental health condition such as bipolar disorder, talk to your specialist as they may want to switch you to an alternative medication which is safe to use during pregnancy. For example: the drug sodium valproate is given to help with epilepsy and bipolar disorder, this drug is teratogenic (can harm a developing baby) so must not be taken if pregnant or trying for a baby. Because of this risk, women using this drug or other drugs known to be harmful in pregnancy are placed on a special Pregnancy Prevention Programme, which is designed to make sure women are aware of the risks and the need to avoid pregnancy. If you are on any medication for depression, it is important to talk to your GP or your psychiatrist about whether it is safe during pregnancy, or whether there might be a better alternative. Don't stop any medication you are taking for a medical condition until you talk with your doctor, as suddenly stopping medication may affect your health. Some medicines can affect sexual performance or sperm quality, so your partner may also need to talk to his doctor if he is taking any medication.

Some common over-the-counter medicines can reduce your chances of conception or increase your risk of miscarriage. For example, ibuprofen, an anti-inflammatory pain-relieving drug, may prevent ovulation, impair fertilization or affect the development of the endometrium. Paracetamol in pregnancy has been used for many years and has been considered safe to use when taken correctly. However, some research is suggesting that this should be reviewed as some studies have shown possible effects on fetal development. *Always* check with the pharmacist that any medicines you buy are safe to take while trying for a baby or when pregnant. Avoid any non-essential treatment. Check that any herbal or alternative remedies or complementary therapies are safe while trying to get pregnant. Ask your doctor, nurse or pharmacist.

Stopping contraception

Once you decide to plan a pregnancy, you will need to think about stopping the contraception you have been using. Many women worry that some methods of contraception, particularly methods that contain hormones (the pill – combined estrogen and progestogen pill and the progestogen-only pill – injection, implant, the skin patch, vaginal ring and the IUS) or the copper IUD will make it difficult to get pregnant when they stop using them. Research is very clear and positive: *no* method of reversible contraception causes infertility.

Using hormonal methods of contraception often results in lighter and less painful periods or 'withdrawal' bleeds. After stopping hormonal contraception your natural periods will return and they may be heavier, redder and more painful due to the extra natural progesterone and thicker endometrium following ovulation. Women often choose hormonal methods to help with 'period' problems and forget the realities of what they were originally like.

Always talk to your doctor or practice nurse if you are concerned about heavy, painful or very long periods, or any bleeding between periods or after sex.

When you stop using contraception your periods and fertility will usually return to normal very quickly. Sometimes ovulation (releasing an egg) can be delayed or be irregular for a short time after stopping hormonal contraception. If you use the contraceptive injection, your periods and fertility may take longer (up to a year or more) to return to normal after stopping the injection. Long-acting reversible methods of contraception (called LARC methods) such as an IUD or IUS or the implant or injectable method of contraception work by protecting you against pregnancy for a long period of time, from a few months to ten years depending on the method. If you are using one of these methods and think you would like a baby in the next year you may choose to switch to a short-acting method such as condoms for a while. This can be a good time to start charting your cycles, have a preconception health check and make any necessary lifestyle modifications. When you are both ready, you can stop using your condoms – being aware of your fertility will help to boost your chances of pregnancy.

You may have heard that it is best to wait three months after stopping hormonal contraception before conceiving, but this is not necessary with today's low-dose hormonal contraception. So, don't worry if you get pregnant very soon after stopping any method of hormonal contraception; this will not harm the baby.

For more information about stopping any method of contraception, you can contact:

- your general practice – ask your doctor or practice nurse
- a contraception or sexual health clinic
- a young people's service such as Brook (there will be an upper age limit).

Past surgery

If you have had any abdominal surgery (e.g. removal of appendix or an ectopic pregnancy), do talk to your doctor about how this may have affected your fertility.

Your partner should talk to his doctor if he has had any injury or surgery to his scrotum (e.g. for undescended testicles; orchitis – inflammation of the testicles – following mumps), or has dilated or varicose veins around his testicles (varicocele). These conditions can affect sperm production.

X-rays and scans

You should not have an x-ray or CT scan (computerized tomography which uses x-rays) while you are pregnant unless it is essential for your health. Ultrasound scans (which use sound waves) are safe during pregnancy as too are MRI scans (magnetic resonance imaging). Always tell your doctor and dentist if you are pregnant or trying for a baby.

Body weight

You can use a calculation to estimate whether your weight is within normal limits for your height. This is known as your body mass index (BMI). Body fat converts androgens (male hormones) into estrogens (female hormones). It also stores estrogen in the typical female fat storage areas: breasts, tummy, thighs and bottom. Body weight and particularly body fat percentage has an important role in female fertility.

Calculate your BMI

BMI is calculated by dividing your body weight in kilograms (kg) by your height in metres squared (see Figure 8.1 for an easy-to-use BMI chart). You can also check your BMI on the Internet or using a BMI phone app.

The ideal BMI associated with normal fertility is in the range of 20–25. Being overweight or underweight can disrupt your periods and severely reduce your chances of conception. If your BMI is more than 27 or less than 19, you may find it more difficult to conceive. The further outside the normal BMI range, the stronger the association with problems with conception, pregnancy and the fetus.

It is important to note that the BMI ranges often quoted relate to a mainly white population; some ethnic groups, such as those of South Asian and Chinese descent, have a lower recommended range of 18–23 because they have a smaller body structure and different body fat distribution.

Overweight

If your BMI is more than 27, this may affect your ovulation and delay conception, so reducing your weight would help. If your BMI is more than 30, you will be medically advised to lose weight before you start trying to conceive. Your doctor may want to check for underlying hormonal problems such as thyroid problems or polycystic ovarian syndrome (PCOS) and to correct any imbalances before you conceive.

Women living with overweight or obesity are more at risk of problems such as diabetes during pregnancy. The higher your BMI is, the higher the risks. Pre-eclampsia, a condition where pregnant women develop high blood pressure, fluid retention and protein in their urine, is more common in overweight women. Although pre-eclampsia is

Weight (kg)	\	\	\	\	\	Height (ft/in)	\	\	\	\	\	\	\	\	\	\	Weight (st/lbs)
	5'0	5'0	5'1	5'2	5'3	5'4	5'4	5'5	5'6	5'7	5'7	5'8	5'8	5'9	5'10	5'11	6'0	
100	43	42	41	40	39	38	37	36	35	35	34	33	32	32	31	30	30	15–10
98	42	41	40	39	38	37	36	36	35	34	33	32	32	31	30	30	29	15–6
96	42	40	39	38	38	37	36	35	34	33	32	32	31	30	30	29	28	15–2
94	41	40	39	38	37	36	35	34	33	33	32	31	30	30	29	28	28	14–11
92	40	39	38	37	36	35	34	33	33	32	31	30	30	29	28	28	27	14–7
90	39	38	37	36	35	34	33	33	32	31	30	30	29	28	28	27	27	14–2
88	38	37	36	35	34	34	33	32	31	30	30	29	28	28	27	27	26	13–12
86	37	36	35	34	34	33	32	31	30	30	29	28	28	27	27	26	25	13–8
84	36	35	35	34	33	32	31	30	30	29	28	28	27	27	26	25	25	13–3
82	35	35	34	33	32	31	30	30	29	28	28	27	26	26	25	25	24	12–13
80	35	34	33	32	31	30	30	29	28	28	27	26	26	25	25	24	24	12–8
78	34	33	32	31	30	30	29	28	28	27	26	26	25	25	24	24	23	12–4
76	33	32	31	30	30	29	28	28	27	26	26	25	25	24	23	23	22	12–0
74	32	31	30	30	29	28	28	27	26	26	25	24	24	23	23	22	22	11–9
72	31	30	30	29	28	27	27	26	26	25	24	24	23	23	22	22	21	11–5
70	30	30	29	28	27	27	26	25	25	24	24	23	23	22	22	21	21	11–0
68	29	29	28	27	27	26	25	25	24	24	23	22	22	21	21	21	20	10–10
66	29	28	27	26	26	25	25	24	23	23	22	22	21	21	20	20	19	10–6
64	28	27	26	26	25	24	24	23	23	22	22	21	21	20	20	19	19	10–1
62	27	26	25	25	24	24	23	22	22	21	21	20	20	20	19	19	18	9–11
60	26	25	25	24	23	23	22	22	21	21	20	20	19	19	19	18	18	9–6
58	25	24	24	23	23	22	22	21	21	20	20	19	19	18	18	18	17	9–2
56	24	24	23	22	22	21	21	20	20	19	19	18	18	18	17	17	17	8–11
54	23	23	22	22	21	21	20	20	19	19	18	18	17	17	17	16	16	8–7
52	23	22	21	21	20	20	19	19	18	18	18	17	17	16	16	16	15	8–3
50	22	21	21	20	20	19	19	18	18	17	17	17	16	16	15	15	15	7–12
48	21	20	20	19	19	18	18	17	17	17	16	16	15	15	15	14	14	7–8
46	20	19	19	18	18	18	17	17	16	16	16	15	15	15	14	14	14	7–3
44	19	19	18	18	17	17	16	16	16	15	15	15	14	14	14	13	13	6–13
42	18	18	17	17	16	16	16	15	15	15	14	14	14	13	13	13	12	6–9
40	17	17	16	16	16	15	15	15	14	14	14	13	13	13	12	12	12	6–4
	1.52	1.54	1.56	1.58	1.60	1.62	1.64	1.66	1.68	1.70	1.72	1.74	1.76	1.78	1.80	1.82	1.84	

Height (m)

Figure 8.1 Body mass index chart: shaded zone indicates the ideal BMI range

usually mild, in rare cases it can cause serious harm to the mother and growth problems in her unborn baby. Women who are overweight are also more likely to miscarry or have a large for dates baby or a stillborn baby. If your BMI is more than 30, your doctor will advise you to take a higher dose (5mg) of folic acid and a vitamin D supplement.

The best way to achieve your ideal weight range and improve your chances of a healthy pregnancy is to combine a healthy diet with exercise (see below). Exercise builds muscle and helps to rebalance your lean-to-fat ratio. Even a modest reduction in weight (around 10 per cent of body weight) will often be enough to improve your hormonal balance and boost your chances of getting pregnant and having a healthy baby.

Underweight

If you are underweight, with a BMI less than 19, your body senses famine and the reproductive system (a non-essential body system) may shut down. This is the body's natural way of knowing it is not safe to become pregnant when so underweight. If you have insufficient body fat to manufacture and store estrogen, this temporarily stops ovulation and your periods may become irregular or stop altogether. This fat store or 'sex fat' is needed to provide the energy for reproduction. If you are underweight, your baby is more likely to be of low birth weight or born prematurely.

You may be within the ideal BMI range, but still not have sufficient stored energy to conceive or hold a pregnancy. If you exercise intensively, you may be too lean (not necessarily underweight as muscle is heavier than fat), and may need to reduce your exercise intensity to boost your chances of conceiving. If you have an eating disorder (anorexia or bulimia) now or have had a problem in the past, you may need advice about how to manage your weight or help your weight increase to improve your chances of conception.

Weight and hormonal contraception

If you are currently using hormonal contraception containing estrogen and progestogen such as the pill, vaginal ring or contraceptive patch, you will have regular bleeding each month. These 'periods' are called hormone 'withdrawal' bleeds. These occur even if you are underweight. This can give you a false impression that all is well. When you stop using these methods, you may find you will not get a period until your weight is within the ideal range for fertility. Try to achieve the ideal BMI range before conceiving, to boost your chances of a healthy pregnancy and healthy baby.

Weight and male fertility

Weight is not so critical for men; however, men who are living with overweight or obesity can have problems caused by excess heat around the testicles. The extra fat cells convert the male hormone testosterone to the female hormone estrogen and reduced testosterone levels may suppress a man's libido and lower his sperm count. If a man is severely underweight such as following serious illness, this can adversely affect his sperm quality.

Managing your weight

If you have not already done so, check your body mass index on the BMI chart (see Figure 8.1). Your GP or practice nurse will be able to advise you on an appropriate diet plan to help you safely and effectively achieve your desired weight range, but the following tips may help:

Tips for losing weight before pregnancy

- Aim for a slow, steady, sustainable weight loss of 0.5–1 kg (1–2 lb) a week.
- You don't need to be at the bottom of the ideal weight range, just within it.
- Eat protein with every meal – nuts, seeds, eggs, fish, chicken, lentils, beans, chickpeas and hummus.
- Always eat breakfast – porridge with fruit, or wholemeal toast and boiled egg.
- Take a homemade salad or lentil and vegetable soup for lunch or choose sandwiches with wholegrain bread, protein and salad.
- Eat a mid-afternoon snack – nuts, seeds, fruit or oatcake with low-fat hummus or cottage cheese.
- Reduce high-fat and processed foods such as ham, sausages, bacon and fast foods (burgers, battered fish, chips).
- Reduce animal and dairy fats (cheese, butter, whole milk). Include skimmed milk and lean meats.

- Eat more fresh fruit and vegetables. High-fibre foods fill you up. Eat vegetables raw, steamed or oven-roasted with olive oil. Limit fruit juices as they are very high in sugar.
- Never skip meals. Eat three meals a day and also a mid-morning, mid-afternoon and bedtime snack.
- Eat good carbohydrates (carbs); these include brown rice, wholegrain pasta, sweet potatoes, butternut squash and wholemeal bread.
- Reduce your portion size. Try eating off a smaller plate.
- Aim for half of your plate to be vegetables, one-quarter protein (lean meat or fish about the size of the palm of your hand) and one-quarter good carbs.
- Avoid eating on the run. Eat slowly and chew your food well.
- Keep junk food and sugary food to a minimum but allow yourself regular treats – like chocolate at the weekend.
- Try plain unsalted popcorn instead of crisps. It's very filling.
- Notice times when you 'comfort eat'. See if there is a pattern: after a hard day at work, a row with your partner, feeling 'empty' or bored.
- Increase your exercise – ensure it fits in with your daily activities and you enjoy it. Walk to the next bus stop, cycle to work, take the stairs – every little helps. Get a fitness tracker and wear footwear that encourages activity. Find an activity you enjoy. Try using a mini-trampoline while watching TV!
- If you have not done any regular exercise for a while, talk to your doctor or practice nurse first.
- Only weigh yourself once a week at most. Some weeks you may lose more weight than others. You will slip up at times, but don't give up completely; just carry on with your healthy eating plan again.
- Don't be tempted to quit if your weight plateaus, as this often means you are now burning fat and increasing your muscle mass. Think about how loose your clothes start to feel.

Tips for gaining weight

- You don't need to start eating junk food; you need calorie- and nutrient-rich meals as this fills you up.
- Make time to shop and to plan meals ahead.
- Avoid artificial sweeteners and diet foods.

- Eat protein with each meal.
- Eat plenty of good carbs for energy.
- Add good fats into your diet – more plant oils from nuts, seeds and avocados and less animal fat.
- Eat plenty of vegetables and oily fish – salmon, mackerel and sardines.
- Nutritious food to help you gain weight, including: avocados, plain nuts, nut butters (peanut, cashew, almond), seeds (pumpkin and sunflower), coconut milk (in curries or smoothies), dried fruits, full-fat hummus, full-fat yoghurt, bananas, wholemeal bread, pasta and rice, sun-dried tomatoes, pesto, sweet potatoes, butternut squash. Use lots of olive oil in salads, for dipping your bread and drizzled on vegetables.
- If you do a lot of exercise, reduce the intensity while still enjoying the positive benefits. About 30 minutes a day is probably a safe limit.

Your lifestyle – impact on fertility, conception and your future child

Eating healthily

Nutritional health passes down through the generations. The egg, from which your life began, developed in one of your mother's ovaries while she was still a fetus inside your grandmother's womb.

Healthy eating is particularly important when preparing for pregnancy, because you are now providing the nourishment for the egg and sperm cells to develop and mature and eventually become your baby. The endometrium also requires vital nutrients to prepare for implantation and to support a healthy pregnancy.

Think about what you eat. Eating a variety of foods, with as much fresh food as possible, helps to ensure that you get all the vitamins and minerals you need.

A healthy balanced diet is made up of protein, carbohydrates and fats. They all play an important role in fertility and pregnancy.

- Protein is essential for growth and repair – protein foods include meat, fish, chicken and eggs; dairy foods such as milk, yogurt and cheese; dairy alternatives such as oat or almond milk; pulses (e.g. peas, beans and lentils), and nuts.

- Carbohydrates for energy – this includes starchy foods (carbohydrates or carbs) such as potatoes, sweet potatoes, bread, pasta, rice and cereals.
- Fruit and vegetables – provide essential vitamins and minerals. Eat at least five portions of fruit and vegetables a day (fresh, dried, frozen, tinned or juiced). Eating a wide variety of colours is the best way to get the full range of nutrients. So, eat the reds, oranges, yellows, blues, and purples as well as your greens – 'eat the rainbow'.
- Fats – 'good' fats are needed for energy and to help the absorption of the fat-soluble vitamins A, D, E and K which are vital for fertility.
- Oily fish – omega-3s. Oily fish such as salmon, mackerel and sardines are rich in omega-3s – docosahexaenoic acid (DHA) and eicosapentaenoic acid (EHA). Some plants are rich in another types of omega-3 fatty acids which the body can convert to DHA and EHA. Good sources of these are flaxseed, chia seeds, walnuts and pumpkin seeds. Omega-3 fatty acids are important for brain function, normal growth and development.
- Drink lots of fluids – water, not sugary drinks.

See below for foods to avoid if pregnant.

Folic acid from food sources

As well as taking your daily supplement of folic acid (see above), eat foods that contain folate, such as dark-green leafy vegetables, pulses (peas, beans and lentils), oats, bread and cereals with added folic acid.

Vitamin D from food sources

Vitamin D, 'the sunshine vitamin', is found in eggs and oily fish such as herring, salmon, mackerel, sardines and tuna. Some foods such as breakfast cereal and bread are fortified with vitamin D. Consider your need for vitamin D supplements (see above).

The following health information is good advice for women trying to get pregnant and for women who know they are pregnant.

Foods to avoid

Severe food poisoning during pregnancy can cause miscarriage, stillbirth or damage to the developing baby. Pregnant women are advised to avoid foods that have a higher risk of causing food poisoning.

The following foods can contain harmful bacteria such as salmonella or listeria. You should avoid them, and any foods made with them, if you are pregnant.

- Unpasteurized milk. Check food labels to make sure milk is pasteurized. All milk sold in supermarkets is pasteurized.
- Soft-cooked or raw eggs that do not have the British Lion stamp that are used in homemade mayonnaise or mousse. Check food labels to make sure eggs are pasteurized. You can use eggs with the British Lion stamp.
- Mould-ripened or soft blue cheeses unless they are *thoroughly* cooked.
- Any cheeses that use unpasteurized milk.
- Undercooked, uncooked or cured meat, including pâté.
- Raw shellfish, such as oysters.

Other foods contain substances that can harm an unborn baby, and you should avoid eating them. These foods are:

- Liver (including liver pâté) because it contains high levels of retinol (the animal form of vitamin A). Similarly avoid vitamin A (retinol) supplements including cod liver oil (see above). However, beta-carotene, the vegetable form of vitamin A is safe and important for fertility. High levels of beta-carotene in the corpus luteum correlate with good progesterone levels. Beta-carotene is found in yellow, red and orange fruits and vegetables and dark-green leafy vegetables.
- Fish such as swordfish, marlin and shark, which can contain high levels of mercury. You can eat tuna, but since it contains some mercury, do not have more than two 140g tins of tuna a week.
- It is safe to eat shellfish provided it has been *thoroughly* cooked. It is also safe to eat sushi provided the fish has been either frozen or smoked first.

Past information suggested that peanuts or foods containing peanuts should be avoided if there is a history of allergy (asthma, eczema, hay fever, food allergy) in your immediate family. This advice has now changed, as the latest research shows no clear evidence of harm. Advice now states that, if you would like to eat peanuts or foods containing peanuts, you can do so as part of a healthy balanced diet unless you have a nut allergy or a health professional advises you not to.

Always check out any questions about food if you are not sure.

Caffeine

Drinks that contain caffeine – coffee, tea (including green tea), cola, energy drinks – and chocolate should be taken in moderation. Too much caffeine can reduce your chance of conception and is also linked to miscarriage and a baby with a low birth weight. Tommy's charity recommends keeping levels of caffeine low to 200 mg per day when planning pregnancy and during pregnancy, which means no more than two small mugs of instant coffee, or one small mug of filter coffee (drink decaffeinated coffee instead), or two small mugs of tea, or one can of cola or energy drink, or two small bars of dark chocolate per day (milk chocolate has half the caffeine of dark). If you have a high caffeine intake, reduce it slowly as symptoms of caffeine withdrawal (headaches, nausea, irritability and fatigue) can be severe in some individuals.

You can find out more information about healthy eating before and during pregnancy by talking to your doctor or nurse or from:

- Tommy's (pregnancy charity)
- Food Standards Agency
- The NHS Eatwell Guide.

Food hygiene

It is important to wash all fruit and vegetables thoroughly. This includes pre-packed salad, fruit and vegetables.

Toxoplasmosis

Toxoplasmosis is an infection caused by a parasite that can live in soil, raw meat and cat faeces. Infection with toxoplasmosis during pregnancy can cause miscarriage, stillbirth, or damage to the baby's eyes, ears or brain.

To reduce the risk of infection, avoid changing cat litter (if you have to do it, wear gloves and wash your hands afterwards), wear gloves when gardening, and wash all soil off fruit and vegetables.

You should also wash your hands thoroughly after handling uncooked meat, and keep uncooked and cooked meat separately from other foods.

Exercise for all

Both you and your partner should start, or keep up, regular exercise when trying to conceive and when pregnant. If you don't exercise, now is a good time to start before you become pregnant. Regular moderate exercise of about 30 minutes a day helps to optimize your weight and improve general health. Exercise also boosts natural endorphins – the 'feel-good' hormones – and helps reduce stress. If you are not used to exercise, start off slowly. The more active and fit you are, the easier it will be for you to cope comfortably with pregnancy.

Physical activity in men stimulates healthy sperm production. Men who are physically active have better-shaped sperm that are stronger swimmers than sedentary men. However, moderation is the key, because men engaged in intensive exercise, such as triathlons, are likely to have less healthy sperm.

Men should avoid anabolic steroids (also sometimes found in protein shakes) as these may affect sperm development.

Walking and swimming are good ways to start getting fit, and a yoga or Pilates class can help with relaxation, posture and muscle tone. Talk to your doctor or exercise instructor if you become pregnant, as you may need to adapt your exercise routine.

Avoid exercise or sports such as martial arts where there is a risk of being hit in the abdomen. Take extra care during activities where there is a risk of falling or losing your balance, such as cycling and horse riding. If you think you may be pregnant, avoid overheating during exercise as this can affect the baby's development in the first 12 weeks. Now is not the time to push yourself to the limit.

Getting fit before you conceive is especially important if you are disabled and use a wheelchair. Regular exercise in preparation for and during pregnancy will improve circulation and help you prepare for the delivery. It helps to prevent constipation and increases strength and flexibility. Talk to your specialist, your GP or a physiotherapist who specializes in women's health about suitable exercises.

You can find out more information and advice about pre-pregnancy exercise, and exercise during pregnancy, from:

- Your general practice – ask your doctor or practice nurse
- Tommy's

- The Royal College of Obstetricians and Gynaecologists (RCOG)
- The Association of Chartered Physiotherapists in Women's Health (ACPWH).

Heat exposure

Your body is designed to incubate a baby at a consistent temperature, so when planning pregnancy and during pregnancy, avoid exposure to additional heat sources (e.g. from hot tubs, saunas or steam rooms). An increase in overall body temperature is linked to neural tube defects such as spina bifida.

Smoking

Stopping smoking is one of the best things you can do to give your baby a healthy start in life and reduce complications in pregnancy and birth. Cigarettes contain tobacco, nicotine and certain chemicals that are harmful for you, your partner and your developing baby. Alternatives such as e-cigarettes (vaping) or nicotine pouches are not thought to be risk-free. We do not know enough about the long-term effects of these products and there is not enough research to show they are safe to use during pregnancy. If you find it difficult to stop smoking, use approved nicotine replacement therapies (NRT) as these have been tested and are recommended instead. If you or your partner smokes, it can reduce your fertility. When pregnant, smoking affects the blood flow through the placenta with potentially serious consequences. Stopping smoking may be the most important thing you can do for your health and the health of your baby. If you both smoke, support each other by giving up together. This will boost your motivation and you are more likely to be successful.

Women who smoke during pregnancy have a greater risk of:

- Miscarriage (loss of a pregnancy before 24 completed weeks)
- Stillbirth (baby born dead after the twenty-fourth completed week of pregnancy)
- Giving birth too early (preterm birth)
- Complications during and after pregnancy and labour
- Having a low-birth-weight baby

- Having a baby with serious birth defects, particularly major gut problems
- Having a child with attention deficit hyperactivity disorder (ADHD).

Babies who have low birth weight or are born prematurely are more likely to have health problems and are at higher risk of sudden infant death syndrome (SIDS, or cot death). The effects of passive smoking (being in an environment where others smoke) can result in poor outcomes for the baby. So, if your partner smokes and you do not, it is important they stop too.

Try not to start smoking again after you've had your baby. Babies whose parents smoke are more likely to suffer from coughs and chest infections, and are at higher risk of SIDS.

Help, support or practical advice on giving up smoking is available from:

- Your general practice – talk to your doctor, practice nurse or midwife
- Your pharmacist
- NHS Smokefree website (and national helpline)
- Tommy's.

Alcohol

Many women ask how much is safe to drink during pregnancy and when preparing for pregnancy. The safest approach is to choose not to drink at all. If you do drink, avoid getting drunk, and try to limit alcohol to the occasional drink. Small amounts of alcohol of 1–2 units not more than once or twice a week have not been shown to be harmful after 12 weeks of pregnancy. However, it is possible that even drinking moderate amounts of alcohol when pregnant can affect a child's future intelligence. Drinking in early pregnancy is likely to be more damaging than later in pregnancy. When a pregnant woman drinks alcohol, the levels of alcohol in her baby's blood rise as high as her own, but because the baby's liver is immature, it can't break down the alcohol as fast as an adult, meaning the baby is exposed to greater amounts of alcohol for longer than the mother.

Drinking heavily (over 6 units a day) before and during pregnancy can affect your ability to conceive and increases your risk of miscarriage, preterm birth, stillbirth, or having a baby of low birth weight. Alcohol can also damage sperm production, so men should cut down on drinking too. Heavy drinking reduces testosterone levels, which can lead to loss of libido, erection difficulties and poor-quality sperm.

If a woman drinks heavily and frequently in pregnancy, or regularly binge drinks (6 or more units of alcohol on any one occasion), this can harm her baby's development and health. Heavy drinking can lead to fetal alcohol syndrome (FAS) and fetal alcohol spectrum disorder (FASD). These describe a range of abnormalities including damage to the facial features, brain, heart and kidneys, and learning difficulties and behavioural problems in later life.

Many pregnancies are unplanned. You may have had a one-off binge (holidays, a party) and then later discover that you conceived at or around this time. Many women worry that this might have caused harm to the baby. It is thought that a single episode of binge drinking is unlikely to be harmful to a woman or her baby.

If you or your partner finds it difficult to cut down on alcohol, you can get help and support from:

- Your general practice – talk to your doctor, nurse or midwife
- Drinkline, the national alcohol helpline
- Drinkaware – a website that can help you count your units, and offers information on drinking in pregnancy and advice on cutting down
- Tommy's

⚠ Did you know?

It takes significantly longer to conceive if a man drinks more than 10–20 units of alcohol per week, smokes more than 15 cigarettes per day, or drinks more than six caffeinated drinks a day.

Alcohol is measured in units. One unit of alcohol is equivalent to half a pint of lager or beer, a small glass of wine or a single shot of spirit. A 750ml bottle of wine is equivalent to 9 units (see Figure 8.2).

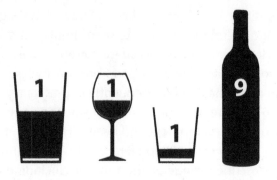

Figure 8.2 What is a unit of alcohol?

Drinks poured at home tend to be larger measures than those in pubs or restaurants. Beer, lager and cider may be ordinary strength, export or extra strong (from 3 to 9 per cent alcohol by volume). A bottle of table wine is about 12 per cent alcohol by volume. Fortified wines may be up to 20 per cent, and spirits are around 40 per cent alcohol.

Recreational drugs

Recreational (illegal) drugs, also known as street drugs, can cause problems with ovulation and irregular periods. Avoid taking them when you are trying to get pregnant and once you are pregnant. Recreational drugs including cannabis, cocaine and amphetamines can seriously affect the developing baby, increasing the chance of low birth weight and some birth defects.

If you inject illegal drugs, see your doctor for referral to help you stop or manage your drug use more safely. Your doctor will also arrange tests for blood-borne infections such as hepatitis B, C and HIV to prevent transmission to your baby. All women who are pregnant are offered HIV and hep B testing on an opt-out basis.

Some women feel anxious that drug use in their past might affect their ability to conceive or damage their unborn baby. There is no evidence of longer-term effects on reproductive health except possibly in the case of very long-term heavy drug use.

Your partner should avoid using recreational drugs too as they can affect sperm quality. Men who frequently use cannabis will have a reduced sperm count and motility (ability to move), which can lead to problems conceiving.

For information on recreational drugs and where to go for help and advice, contact Frank (see Resources).

Workplace, home and environmental hazards

All of us are exposed every day to environmental chemicals – where we live, work or play. Mostly they are safe, but research is not available addressing the cumulative affects they may have and this is certainly true with regard to any risks that might affect fertility or pregnant women and their babies. As such, the general advice is to be more aware of what we do or eat, take appropriate precautions and, when in doubt, check.

Some workplace occupations can expose you to substances (e.g. radiation, chemicals, solvents, paint fumes, fungicides and pesticides) or surroundings (e.g. heat exposure, air quality, noise, vibrations) that may be harmful if you become pregnant or cause difficulties when trying to get pregnant. If you are concerned, speak to your manager, personnel officer, or health and safety officer to find out more about any risks. Always wear any protective clothing supplied by your employer.

Your partner also has the right to a safe working environment. Heat exposure for men is important to consider as a man's testicles hang outside his body at a temperature of about two degrees below normal body temperature. When scrotal temperature rises, sperm production may be compromised. Sitting for long periods of time, whether driving as an occupation or sitting at a desk all day, can increase scrotal temperature. Your partner's clothing is important too he should avoid wearing tight-fitting underwear or jeans. He should also avoid additional exposure to heat, such as having long hot baths.

Physical and psychological stress is possibly the main hazard at work. Work stress can cause short or irregular menstrual cycles and delay conception. Make sure you (and your partner) try to manage your work environment. Take a proper lunch break. Leave work on time. Now is a good time to consider your work–life balance.

For more information and advice on rights in the workplace, including mental health at work and protective measures against the spread of COVID-19 in enclosed spaces, see the Health and Safety Executive website (see Resources).

Stress

Life can be stressful, and undoubtedly trying for a baby can be physically and emotionally demanding. But the question as to whether stress contributes to or causes delays in conception is controversial – some say stress reduces your chance of conception, but other studies do not find a link.

Stress is really any situation you perceive as threatening or challenging. This may be a physical threat, but also includes things like overwork, exhaustion or grief. The stress may be internal or external, within or outside your control. You may feel internal stress if you fail to achieve a goal such as getting pregnant. You may experience external stress through pressures from relatives, or seeing pregnant friends.

When you experience stress, your body turns on the 'fight or flight' response. The hormone adrenaline increases your heart rate and breathing rate, diverts blood flow to your large muscles, slows down digestion and inhibits reproduction. If a lion is chasing you, it is no time to be digesting food, making sperm or ovulating.

Stress may reduce your daily chances of conception during your fertile time. You may have irregular cycles, ovulation may not occur, or you may have a short luteal phase with insufficient time for implantation. Some women under stress have normal menstrual cycles, but still fail to conceive until the stress is alleviated.

Long-term chronic stress can impact on your quality of life, suppress your immune system and delay conception. If you are working long hours and stressed by the pressures of life, this is not conducive to your body taking on a long-term 'stressful' project – that of pregnancy, breastfeeding and nurturing a child.

Interestingly research shows that stress is unlikely to affect the outcome of IVF. So, although fertility treatment can be stressful, you can be reassured that feeling anxious or worried because of fertility delays or treatments, this is unlikely to further reduce your chances of pregnancy.

If you feel stressed, try to find the encouragement and support you need to help you modify the way you respond to stress. Talk to your partner or friend; or ask your GP to refer you for counselling or cognitive behaviour therapy. Exercise can be a great stress-buster.

Some complementary therapies can also be very relaxing and may help manage stress. Mindfulness strategies can be very helpful. For more information on this, see the mental health section on the NHS website (see Resources).

Sexual and relationship problems

If you are feeling anxious about getting pregnant or concerned about delays in conception, then it is a great time to start trying to take control of the sexual side of your relationship. Although it can be helpful to understand your menstrual cycle and your fertile time, this can put added pressure on your sexual relationship. If spontaneity is lost and lovemaking becomes too focused around penetration and ejaculation, then sex becomes mechanical and your relationship may start to suffer.

A baby will not solve a relationship problem. Having a baby puts a strain on even the healthiest relationship. The birth of the first child and the transition to parenthood is possibly the single greatest challenge to any individual or couple.

If you have any sexual or relationship problems, now is the time to try to sort them out before you get pregnant. For further help, contact Relate or the College of Sexual and Relationship Therapists (COSRT) (see Resources).

Travel

Travel can disrupt your attempts to conceive. If, for example, you or your partner has to travel with work, try to calculate your fertile time and avoid travelling during this time if possible. You can learn to identify your fertile time, but if you are travelling extensively then this can temporarily disrupt your cycles.

Air travel

Some women are concerned about flying when trying to conceive because of the atmospheric changes inside the plane: the decrease in air pressure, reduced humidity and slight increase in radiation. Occasional flights are not considered to present a significant risk during pregnancy or when trying to conceive. If your pregnancy is straightforward, there is no evidence that flying is harmful to you or your baby. If you are a member of a flight crew or fly frequently as part of your work, you should seek additional advice from your occupational health department or your doctor. Body scanners used for security checks are safe to use when pregnant.

The risk of deep vein thrombosis (DVT) is increased during pregnancy and for six weeks after birth. This is nature's protective mechanism to reduce excessive postnatal bleeding. Long flights (defined as more than four hours) in cramped conditions also increase the risk of DVT, so if you think you could be pregnant:

- Try to get an aisle seat and move around and do some exercise every 30 minutes
- Wear flight socks (if already pregnant use properly fitted graduated elastic compression stockings)
- Drink water at regular intervals, but avoid alcohol or fizzy drinks or drinks containing caffeine as these are dehydrating.

Most women can safely travel by air during pregnancy provided that they have no pregnancy complications and have had a check-up with their doctor. The best time to travel is between 14 and 28 weeks of pregnancy when there is a lower risk of miscarrying or going into labour. In the first 12 weeks of pregnancy, all women are at some risk of miscarriage. There is no evidence to suggest that flying increases your risk of miscarriage; however, many women prefer to avoid flying in early pregnancy, particularly if they have miscarried in the past, are older, or have taken a while to conceive. Check with your airline about their rules on pregnant passengers before you book. If your pregnancy is over 28 weeks, the airline will ask you to get a letter from your doctor or midwife stating when your baby is due and confirming that you are not at risk of any complications. Some airlines will allow you to fly beyond the recommended time.

Talk to your doctor about any travel plans and get up-to-date information from a specialist travel clinic about what travel vaccinations or pills (such as anti-malarial tablets) can or should not be used. Also find out what and where the medical facilities are at your destination in the event of miscarriage, ectopic pregnancy or premature labour. Make sure you are insured and take your pregnancy notes with you.

Pregnant women or women trying to get pregnant should avoid travelling to areas where there is a risk of malaria or the Zika virus. Both malaria and the Zika virus are spread by mosquitos. The Zika virus infection is spread by day-biting mosquitos. A number of cases of sexual transmission of the Zika virus have been reported. The Zika virus infection can result in serious birth defects. As such travel advice should be obtained four to six weeks before travelling to a country with this virus. The general advice is that women who are pregnant or women planning to become pregnant should not go to countries with the Zika virus. Women should not become pregnant in areas with active Zika virus transmission. If you or your partner have been in a country infected with the Zika virus, use effective contraception and talk to your doctor before you try for a baby; the general advice is to delay getting pregnant for a minimum of three months after leaving the country. See information from National Travel Health Network (NaTHNaC) (see Resources).

Employment rights

Your doctor can advise you about employment rights and maternity benefits. It is unlawful sex discrimination for an employer to treat a woman less favourably because she intends to get pregnant or is going through IVF. You are entitled to paid time-off for antenatal appointments. If you are having IVF, you are only entitled to paid time off after embryo transfer. Find out about pregnancy and maternity rights in the workplace from Maternity Action (see Resources).

Disability aspects

If you have a disability, you may need to consider the practical and medical feasibility of having a baby and looking after a child. Concentrate on what you will be able to do as a parent, rather than what you won't be able to do. Think about the practical support you can expect from your partner or family and any additional support or appliances you may need. You will also need to consider whether there is any medical risk to the child or yourself because of your disability. Talk with your doctor or specialist before you get pregnant, so you feel confident about planning a pregnancy.

Some disabilities occur in families – that is, they have a genetic origin – and if this is the case your doctor can refer you to a genetic counsellor and/or specialist, who will discuss the probability of having a child with this disability. Knowing whether this might occur will allow you to consider all your options.

There are few disabilities that affect a woman's fertility directly, but some drugs used to manage a disability can affect the menstrual cycle or sperm production, so discuss your medication and plans to conceive with your doctor. If you or your partner have a disability, which make sex challenging or penetration not possible, you can be referred to an appropriate specialist for further help and advice. The College of Sexual and Relationship Therapists also provides good information and support (see Resources).

Having a disability does not mean you cannot, or should not, become pregnant, but you may need more support and advice than someone without any disability. If you become pregnant, speak to your doctor as soon as possible. If your disability requires consultant-led care, you may require specialist advice about pregnancy. You can also request that your maternity care is provided by the hospital at which your consultant is based.

For more information on pregnancy and planning a pregnancy when you have a disability, contact the organization Disability Pregnancy and Parenthood (see Resources).

Timing sex to optimize your chances

The accepted guidance on timing intercourse to conceive is to have sex every two to three days throughout the whole menstrual cycle. This optimizes sperm health and ensures that sex coincides with the full width of the woman's fertile time. A man needs to ejaculate every two to three days (whether through intercourse or masturbation) to maintain a plentiful supply of fresh healthy sperm. If he does not ejaculate for more than four to five days, his sperm quality deteriorates and it takes two ejaculations to clear through the poorer-quality sperm. For practical purposes, it is not always possible to have intercourse every couple of days, which is why it helps to be aware of the fertile time in your cycle (see Chapter 3)

Using fertility awareness to conceive

The information below summarizes what you need to know to time intercourse to increase your chances of pregnancy.

- You can get a rough idea of your fertile time based on your past cycle lengths – use both the shortest and longest cycle calculations to find the widest possible window when sex could lead to pregnancy (Chapter 3) and aim to have intercourse every couple of days throughout this time
- Within your calculated fertile time, the changes in cervical secretions give the best indication of the days when sperm could survive in your body waiting to meet the egg.
- You could conceive from intercourse on *any* day you notice secretions, but the days with the wetter, transparent, slippery, stretchy secretions have the highest chance of pregnancy (Chapter 3).
- Intercourse on peak day (the *last* day of wetter, slippery, transparent secretions) carries the highest chance of pregnancy, but the day with the most profuse secretions is a really good day too – this is often one or two days before peak.

Figure 8.3 shows changes in the cervical secretions. Notice that the fertile time starts on the first day of any secretions. Peak day is the last day of highly fertile secretions, and the fertile time ends three days after peak. You can download a blank chart to record a series of cycles from the FertilityUK website (see Appendix)

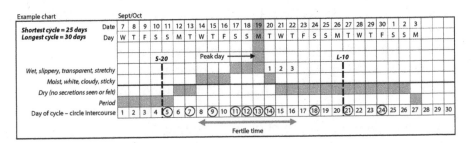

Figure 8.3 Chart showing intercourse timing to optimize chances of conception

The cervical secretions will vary in amount and quality and this is normal, but there are some specific factors which may disrupt the pattern of secretions, or make it more difficult to distinguish the changes (see Chapter 3).

Does it help to chart temperature?

Temperature charting will not help you to time sex to conceive, but it may give you more information about your cycles and help to reassure you that you are ovulating. If you wish to take your temperature, you will find details on how to record an accurate temperature (Chapter 3). It is important not to get stressed by taking daily temperatures – it can be counterproductive – but you may find it useful to chart your temperature for a few cycles.

Temperature can be used to confirm pregnancy: if you have 20 days or more of high temperatures, it is highly likely that you are pregnant. You may notice a second rise in temperature (often to around 37 °C) about a week after the ovulation rise, giving a tri-phasic pattern (see Figure 3.10), but not all women will see this – it is the sustained rise that indicates pregnancy – this can be confirmed by a pregnancy test.

Temperature charts help to confirm ovulation. A biphasic chart with ten or more high temperatures confirms that ovulation is likely to have occurred in that cycle. It also confirms that that there is sufficient time for implantation. If you have three or more consecutive cycles with short luteal phases (fewer than ten high temperatures) or monophasic cycles (with no temperature rise), this requires further investigation. Your GP may suggest hormone tests including a progesterone test to confirm ovulation (see below).

Does the fertility chart show anything else?

Recording your cycles can help to identify changes which may make it more difficult to conceive. For example, it is common to have slight spotting just before your period starts, but if you have *more than* two days of spotting, this could affect implantation or be a sign of a gynaecological problem (see Chapter 3). Increasing your awareness of changes in your cervical secretions helps you to recognize what is a normal pattern (in terms of quantity and quality of secretions); it also helps you to detect the first signs of an abnormal discharge (see Chapter 3).

What about ovulation predictor kits?

Ovulation predictor kits and other fertility gadgets are widely available through pharmacies and the Internet – they are often aggressively marketed and give the impression that technology is the only way to find your most fertile time. If you are aware of your cervical secretions, then there is no advantage to using these kits – best to save your money; however, if you are struggling to identify the changes in your secretions, then one of the simple ovulation predictor kits (which test hormones in urine) may help (see Chapter 3).

Are there any disadvantages to charting?

There is a fine balance here between the benefits of being aware of your fertile time and the tensions that can result if this starts to dictate how and when to have sex. Men find it particularly difficult if the whole bedroom is turned into a laboratory with thermometers, ovulation predictor kits and goodness knows what other gizmos lying around. The key to conception is frequent sex, not 'perfect' timing.

Frequency of ejaculation

It takes about 70 days for a sperm to be produced, but as sperm production is a continuous process there are always plenty of fully mature sperm at any one time. Daily ejaculation may reduce the volume of seminal fluid and the total sperm count, but it improves the sperm motility and genetic quality, so it may actually boost chances of pregnancy. Having regular intercourse every two to three days should provide more than enough healthy sperm to fertilize an egg.

Sexual position

Many women ask about the best position to have sex to optimize conception. There is no 'best' position. Provided that your partner is ejaculating deep inside your vagina, the sperm will sort out the rest. So, the best position is whatever position you and your partner enjoy and feel comfortable with. Sex should be passionate, varied and fun. Some women who have a retroverted (backwards pointing) uterus (see Chapter 2) may find some sexual positions more uncomfortable but there is no evidence that any particular sexual position improves chances of pregnancy.

'Flow-back'

Many women trying to conceive get anxious about losing seminal fluid after sex. When the semen is first ejaculated, it is a creamy-white colour and designed to stick to the cervix. Within a few minutes, the seminal fluid liquefies and becomes colourless. During this process, the sperm are released and they start their journey towards the egg. Most of the fluid lost from your vagina in the 'flow-back' is seminal fluid with dead or dying sperm. The strong healthy swimmers should be well on their way.

'Good' sex and 'bad' sex

It is not always easy to keep the passion alive, particularly if you have been trying to conceive for a while, so try to be creative and think about how you can get the intimacy back into your relationship. Mechanical 'baby-making' sex is pretty dull and not conducive to conception, and it will certainly not make either of you keen to repeat the exercise. If sex becomes a chore, you will inevitably end up having less sex, so the best sex is anything that encourages you to want to have more sex (see section on sexual response in Chapter 2).

Sexual difficulties

If you have any sexual difficulties that make penetration painful, or your partner suffers from problems with erections or ejaculation, a specially trained counsellor may be able to help you. Sexual difficulties are remarkably common and not something to be embarrassed about. Talk to your doctor or practice nurse or contact Relate (see Resources).

Lubricants

Almost all water-based and oil-based lubricants affect sperm motility (ability to move) under laboratory conditions. Saliva also damages sperm as it contains digestive enzymes, so be careful with oral sex if you are trying to conceive. If you need a lubricant, then logically a lubricant that is advertised as 'non-spermicidal' should be okay, but that just means that it does not contain a spermicidal component which kills sperm. Pre-Seed and Conceive Plus are the only lubricants which do not have an adverse effect on sperm motility, but it is still not known whether they could affect sperm DNA.

Self-insemination

Self-insemination offers a low-tech method of conceiving when intercourse is not possible. It is commonly used by single women and lesbian couples, but it also provides an alternative for straight couples who are experiencing sexual difficulties.

Collecting the seminal fluid

At ejaculation, 2–5 ml of seminal fluid is ejaculated in a series of five to ten spurts, often with a pelvic thrust in between. When first released, the fluid is creamy-white, thick and sticky. After a few minutes, it starts to liquefy. The volume of fluid depends partly on the time since the previous ejaculation. Although there may be a higher volume after a longer interval, the sperm quality will not be so good. For optimum sperm quality, a man should ejaculate every two to three days.

You will need a collection pot and a plastic syringe or pipette. These can be obtained from most chemists. All equipment should be sterile and for single use. Self-insemination kits are also available from Andrology Solutions (see Resources).

- Ask your partner to masturbate into the collection pot – try to collect the whole ejaculate.
- Wait for about ten minutes until the seminal fluid liquefies.
- Draw the fluid up by squeezing the bulb of the pipette (or drawing up the plunger of the syringe).

The insemination

- Use a finger to guide the pipette (or syringe) into the vagina as far as is comfortable.
- Squeeze the pipette to release the contents in one go (to mimic ejaculation) deep in the vagina. If using a syringe, use the plunger to deposit the fluid in one go.
- Ideally try and masturbate to orgasm during the insemination – this encourages the muscular uterine contractions to help suck the sperm through the cervical opening.
- Try to lie flat for ten to 15 minutes to keep the sperm in contact with the cervix.

Aim to make the insemination process as intimate as you can – your partner may wish to do the inseminations and you can help each other to achieve orgasm. Ideally an insemination should be performed almost immediately after the fluid has been produced but, if necessary, it can be kept for a few hours in the pipette or syringe (at body temperature). It should not be allowed to dry out.

Complementary therapies

Complementary therapies are sometimes described as alternative medicine. However, 'complementary' better describes these therapies, as they should always be used alongside, but never replace, the treatment offered by your doctor. Complementary therapies include a wide range of disciplines. Most of these are not regulated, and some therapies have more evidence to support their use than others. The most commonly used therapies are acupuncture, herbal treatments, homeopathy, reflexology, hypnotherapy and massage.

Acupuncture is possibly the therapy most closely associated with fertility. Many women (and men) benefit from the stress reduction effects of acupuncture, but it is unclear whether acupuncture improves the conception rate for couples trying naturally or with IVF. For registered acupuncturists, see the British Acupuncture Council (see Resources).

Do not take any herbal remedies, as these are unlicensed products with little or no information on their safety immediately before or during pregnancy. If you want to use any complementary therapies, talk to your doctor about this and make sure that you see a qualified and registered practitioner.

Get on and enjoy life

The most difficult thing about trying to conceive can be the uncertainty about if and when pregnancy will happen. Until now, if you have wanted something badly enough; you have probably figured out a way to make it happen. But now you may be at a loss as to how to achieve this thing that others seem to find so easy. The sense of being out of control can feel frightening.

Reproduction, rather like the digestive system, is not under conscious control. The big thing about trying to conceive is to just let it happen – to focus on other things in life. A relaxing holiday can be great; try to get a good work–life balance and make an effort to get out and enjoy life. This is often precisely the time when pregnancy happens – when you 'forget to think about it'. If you conceive unintentionally and have not made any lifestyle changes – don't panic. Generations of women have produced strong healthy babies under all sorts of adverse conditions without any preconception planning, so relax.

There are essentially only two things most couples need to achieve pregnancy – the first thing is sex and the second is time (and it can take a lot of both). Women often feel anxious knowing that they only have a few days during each cycle when they could conceive; whereas men tend to be more laid-back about it, knowing that they have a constant supply of sperm and a quiet confidence that it will happen in its own time. Try not to think of this as 'Project Baby'. The trick is to distract yourself as much as possible and to get on with things, enjoying life rather than putting it on hold.

When you get a positive pregnancy test (see above), you are likely to be really excited. However, if you have miscarried in the past, you may also start to feel anxious. Whether this is your first pregnancy or a subsequent pregnancy, now is the time to book your appointment with your GP or your midwife to discuss your antenatal care, arrange your first scan and discuss any concerns.

9

Fertility concerns and delays

Even if you have made all the lifestyle changes, kept track of your cycles and been having sexual intercourse two to three times a week, it may still take a while to get pregnant. Many factors affect fertility and conception, so don't be surprised or upset if you do not get pregnant straight away. It often takes much longer, and this is normal. You may want to consider a few things to make sure you are still on track.

After contraception

For many years you may have been using contraception conscientiously to avoid pregnancy, fearing that a slip-up could lead to pregnancy. If you experience a delay in conception, you start to hear the other side of the same story – which is that it takes on average about six months to conceive. It's all about statistics. Remember, no reversible method of contraception causes infertility, although temporary delays may occur with some methods.

After abortion

If you have made the difficult decision to have an abortion in the past, then this may affect your feelings if you now face a fertility delay. Abortion (medical or surgical abortion) is a very safe procedure and will not affect your chances of conceiving again provided there were no serious infections or injuries to your uterus or cervix. If you had any complications after your abortion, or if you feel distressed about a past abortion, talk to your doctor or practice nurse.

If you are having difficulties conceiving and have previously had an abortion due to fetal abnormality, possibly at a later stage in pregnancy, then the same medical information applies. This can be very difficult to cope with emotionally, so talk to your doctor and consider seeing a fertility counsellor.

After miscarriage

Miscarriage is very common (see below). Although some women will conceive very quickly after miscarrying, it is not unusual for it to take several months for fertility to return and your body to be ready physically and emotionally to cope with another pregnancy. There is no definite 'right' time to try for another pregnancy after a miscarriage. Understandably, many women hope they will quickly become pregnant again, anticipating that it will feel easier to cope emotionally. However, it is not unusual to be unable to conceive again until after the due date. After experiencing a difficult time around their expected date of delivery, many women say they feel 'different', somehow more 'back to normal' and conception follows. If you have had a late miscarriage or your baby was stillborn, then it can take longer for your body to recover physically and for you to be emotionally ready to conceive again. Your body has a remarkable way of suppressing fertility in an effort to protect you from further trauma until it seems you are coping with life again. If you have not conceived one year after a miscarriage, then talk to your doctor or practice nurse.

After childbirth

If you have had a baby and are planning another pregnancy, it takes a while for your body to recover from pregnancy and childbirth. It is generally advisable to try to have a gap of about two years between one birth and the next to optimize your own health and that of a future baby; however, if you are older (over 35), then age is not on your side and it may be advisable to try to conceive again sooner.

Breastfeeding acts as a natural contraceptive – it suppresses fertility. Although it is possible to conceive while you are still breastfeeding, it is less likely if you are fully (or almost fully) breastfeeding and your periods have not returned (or are not yet regular again). Some women are unable to conceive again until they have *completely* stopped breastfeeding. If you are not breastfeeding, fertility normally returns very quickly after childbirth. (For more detailed information about fertility after childbirth, see Chapter 6.)

If you have been trying for another baby and you have not become pregnant, it may be useful to consider:

- Has anything changed health-wise since the birth of your last baby?
- Have you completely stopped breastfeeding?
- Have your breasts returned to normal (soft without any leakage)?
- Have your menstrual cycles returned? Do they seem normal for you?
- Has your weight changed significantly since your last conception?
- Has anything changed health-wise for your partner?
- Do you have the same or a different partner?
- Are you having regular sexual intercourse?
- Were there any problems with your last pregnancy, birth or postnatal recovery?

If you have any concerns about your health or about your fertility after childbirth, talk to your doctor or practice nurse.

Why it may take longer to conceive

The main causes of fertility problems are male factor problems, disorders of ovulation, damaged tubes, and disorders of the uterus or pelvis. Many factors can affect the delicate balance of reproduction. In almost half of the couples with fertility delays, there are problems with both partners. In about a quarter of all couples, there will be no cause identified (unexplained). It can be most frustrating to hear that there is no obvious cause for delayed conception. IVF may be suggested in some cases of 'unexplained' infertility. The aim with IVF is to help you get pregnant, but sometimes the IVF process itself helps to identify a possible cause. The intensive monitoring through IVF may highlight defects with the egg or sperm, the fertilization rate or embryo quality, or problems with the endometrium and implantation.

Are you ovulating?

One possible problem is that ovulation may not occur every cycle. If you have recently stopped hormonal contraception, ovulation may be delayed or irregular for a few cycles. If you have been using a contraceptive injection, ovulation may be delayed or irregular for up to a year. If you are over 35, under- or overweight, or very stressed, this can also affect ovulation.

There are only three ways to confirm ovulation conclusively: being pregnant (the best possible proof), a raised progesterone level (midway through the luteal phase) or a scan showing a collapsed follicle. An ovulation predictor kit identifies a surge in luteinizing hormone (the trigger for ovulation) and is a good sign, but it does not prove ovulation has occurred. Similarly, wetter cervical secretions are a good sign (showing high estrogen levels) but they do not prove ovulation. If you are concerned you may not be ovulating, see your doctor.

A period does not prove you are ovulating.

If you ovulate (release an egg), it's simple – you either conceive or you don't. So, within the next two weeks, only one of two things can happen: *either* you get a period – so you are not pregnant; *or* you don't get a period and a pregnancy test shows you are pregnant.

If you don't ovulate, after a certain time your hormone levels will drop anyway and you will get a bleed – technically this is a 'hormone withdrawal bleed'. While this is not a 'true period' it is not possible to tell the difference, although some women may feel that their 'period' is lighter than usual. There can be exceptions, such as for women who continue to get 'periods' (episodes of light vaginal bleeding) throughout pregnancy, but this is uncommon.

Is there enough time for implantation?

Even if there are sperm waiting for the egg to be released, you may not become pregnant in the first few months of trying. Sometimes fertilization takes place but the egg does not implant securely. If you are monitoring your cervical secretions and notice that the time from your peak day until your next period is consistently less than ten days, then this may indicate a problem with implantation and you should talk to your doctor.

Is your partner producing good-quality sperm?

There may be a problem with the number or quality of your partner's sperm. Sperm production can be damaged by a number of factors (e.g. heat – see Chapter 2 – and lifestyle factors including smoking and alcohol – see Chapter 8). If your partner has previously fathered a child or had a pregnancy with you or a previous partner, this does not necessarily mean that he is still producing healthy sperm. Your GP can arrange a sperm test.

The great sperm race

- Over 100 million sperm are deposited in the vagina.
- Only a few thousand sperm enter the fallopian tubes.
- Around 100 sperm will surround the egg.
- Just one sperm will fertilize the egg.
- The winning sperm will have lashed its tail around 20,000 times.

Your age

A woman's age is possibly the most significant factor predicting fertility potential. Your chances of conception decrease, as you get older (notably after 35) as the quantity and quality of eggs deteriorate with age.

A woman is born with her lifetime supply of eggs – approximately 1–2 million immature eggs. During reproductive life, approximately 300–400 mature eggs are released at ovulation and the remainder are lost through natural cell death. The rate at which these eggs are lost varies between women, and this largely explains the difference in age at menopause.

A man's fertility is affected by age too, but to a much lesser extent. Men continue to produce sperm into old age; however, from around 40, a man's sperm quality starts to deteriorate, leading to a longer time to conception and an increased risk of miscarriage.

Age at menopause

Most women reach menopause in their early 50s. Some women will have irregular and often short cycles approaching the menopause, but other women's cycles remain regular and then suddenly stop. A woman's fertility ceases up to ten years before she has her final period, which means that, if you were going to have your final period at the age of 51 (average age), you could be infertile after about 41. Women may go on having periods and noticing changes in the cervical secretions for a number of years after they stop ovulating. Some women have a later menopause so could conceive well into their forties, but other women have an earlier menopause or even a premature menopause (before 40 years) so they would be infertile from a much younger age.

Declining egg quality

As the number of eggs age and decline, so too does the quality, resulting in more chromosomally abnormal eggs. This decline is marked after about 35 years when the pregnancy rate falls and the miscarriage rate increases. The incidence of chromosomal disorders such as Down's syndrome increases with age. In Down's syndrome (also known as Trisomy 21) the baby inherits an extra chromosome 21.

! Age conundrum

- It can take longer and be more difficult to get pregnant if you are over 35.
- A woman will usually go on having 'periods' long after her fertility has ended.
- 'Fertile' secretions are commonly seen long after natural fertility has ended.
- Older women have significantly lower success rates with IVF.
- While many women over 35 have healthy pregnancies and babies, miscarriages and problems with pregnancy and childbirth are more frequent than with younger women.
- Many older women who become pregnant have used donor eggs, or in some cases have used their own eggs which they froze when they were younger.
- The time approaching menopause is very unpredictable. Women who do not wish to get pregnant must use a reliable contraceptive method for two years after their final period if under 50 and for one year if over 50.

Home test kits to check fertility potential

There are a number of kits on the market designed to test a couple's fertility potential. Very basic sperm tests check sperm concentration and motility. They do not test sperm morphology (shape) or identify problems such as anti-sperm antibodies or problems with the seminal fluid. Similarly, home kits which test a woman's FSH level can give misleading results and false reassurance.

When to seek help

If you are worried that it is taking an unusually long time to conceive, always talk to your doctor. Sometimes reassurance is all that is needed. Because some couples do take longer than others to conceive, many doctors prefer you to have been having regular sex, two to three times a week without contraception, for at least a year, before referring you for fertility tests. If you are over 35, or if you have any known medical or fertility problems, you may be referred for help after six months.

⧵ Remember

- Around 80–90 out of 100 couples become pregnant within one year
- Around 95 out of 100 couples become pregnant within two years.
- If you don't get pregnant at once, you are not unusual and it doesn't necessarily mean that you have a problem.

What to expect from your GP when attending with fertility concerns

If you have not already seen your GP when you were at the planning stages, then he or she will still want to do the basic preconception health checks. These may include checking your rubella status (see Chapter 8) as well as carrying out simple fertility tests and possibly referring you to a fertility clinic for further investigations.

Blood test to confirm ovulation

Your GP will arrange a blood test to confirm ovulation. This is often referred to as the 'day 21 progesterone test' – the blood test needs to be timed for midway through your luteal phase – so that would only be day 21 if you have a regular 28-day cycle. You can time the test more accurately by arranging the test for about six days after your temperature rise or seven days after peak day. Provided your period starts about a week after the test was taken, you will know that it was accurately timed.

Depending on your progesterone results, your GP may check other reproductive hormones (FSH, LH, estrogen) in the first few days of your cycle. Your GP may also check your thyroid hormones, prolactin and testosterone and do a full blood count (to exclude anaemia) – particularly if your cycles are irregular.

Semen analysis

At the same time as checking your hormones, your GP will arrange a semen analysis (sperm test) for your partner. Make sure your partner follows the instructions carefully. He will normally be asked to abstain from any sexual activity (including masturbation) for two to five days before test day – this is to help standardize the test. If the results of the first semen analysis are abnormal, a repeat test is usually done three months later to allow time for a new batch of sperm to be made. In some circumstances, the test is repeated sooner.

What to expect at the fertility clinic

Fertility clinics provide specialist help in gynaecology and women's reproductive health care. At your first visit, the gynaecologist will look at your preliminary test results and discuss the need for further blood tests and fertility investigations.

Ovarian reserve tests

One of the first things to determine is your ovarian reserve – this gives an idea of the approximate number of eggs left in your ovaries and whether this is normal for your age. Anti-mullerian hormone (AMH) is produced by the small antral (resting) follicles, each of which contains an immature egg. You may also have a pelvic ultrasound (internal) scan to determine the number of antral follicles – this is your antral follicle count (AFC). The results of these two tests are used to determine how your ovaries might respond to fertility drugs and to predict your chances of success with assisted conception. Age remains the key factor: younger women have a higher chance of pregnancy, even if they have a reduced ovarian reserve.

Fertility investigations

During an ultrasound scan, the gynaecologist or sonographer checks for conditions such as polycystic ovaries (a hormonal imbalance with many small cysts in the ovaries). A scan may also identify an abnormally shaped uterus, fibroids (benign growths in the uterus) or polyps (benign growths in the uterus or cervix). Fibroids and polyps are not cancerous, but they may cause problems with conception, implantation or a developing pregnancy.

Provided your partner has good-quality sperm, you may have a dye put through your uterus and tubes to check the tubes are open, healthy and clear of any blockages. The dye test may be an x-ray with dye – hystero-salpingogram (HSG) – or ultrasound with dye – hysterosalpingo-contrast sonography (HyCoSy). If you have a history of pelvic surgery or pelvic symptoms such as severe pain during your periods or deep pain during intercourse, you may require a laparoscopy. This is a keyhole procedure performed under general anaesthetic in which a gynaecologist inserts a small telescope through your belly button to explore the pelvis and to see whether dye can be passed through your tubes. Conditions such as endometriosis or adhesions (scar tissue) may be diagnosed during laparoscopy and they can be treated at the same time. Figure 9.1 shows the sequence in which fertility tests and investigations are likely to be carried out.

Fertility treatments

Depending on the outcome of your fertility investigations, you may be offered treatment. This ranges from correcting hormonal imbalances, to stimulating your ovaries with a fertility drug such as clomiphene, through to assisted conception treatments such as intra-uterine insemination (IUI) or in-vitro fertilization (IVF). Sometimes it is necessary to inject the sperm into the egg during IVF; this is known as intra-cytoplasmic sperm injection, or ICSI.

If you do not have a male partner, or your partner has azoospermia (no sperm) or serious abnormalities with his semen analysis, then donor

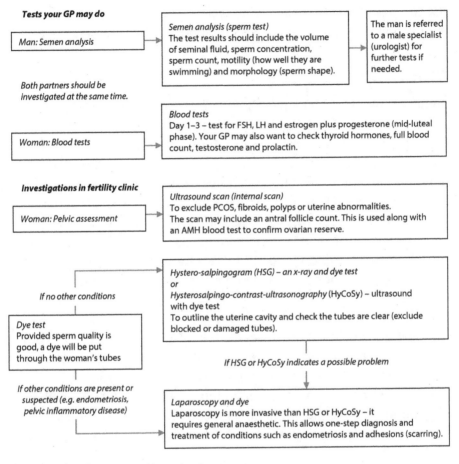

Tests your GP may do

Man: Semen analysis → Semen analysis (sperm test)
The test results should include the volume of seminal fluid, sperm concentration, sperm count, motility (how well they are swimming) and morphology (sperm shape). → The man is referred to a male specialist (urologist) for further tests if needed.

Both partners should be investigated at the same time.

Woman: Blood tests → Blood tests
Day 1–3 – test for FSH, LH and estrogen plus progesterone (mid-luteal phase). Your GP may also want to check thyroid hormones, full blood count, testosterone and prolactin.

Investigations in fertility clinic

Woman: Pelvic assessment → Ultrasound scan (internal scan)
To exclude PCOS, fibroids, polyps or uterine abnormalities. The scan may include an antral follicle count. This is used along with an AMH blood test to confirm ovarian reserve.

If no other conditions → Hystero-salpingogram (HSG) – an x-ray and dye test
or
Hysterosalpingo-contrast-ultrasonography (HyCoSy) – ultrasound with dye test
To outline the uterine cavity and check the tubes are clear (exclude blocked or damaged tubes).

Dye test
Provided sperm quality is good, a dye will be put through the woman's tubes

If HSG or HyCoSy indicates a possible problem

If other conditions are present or suspected (e.g. endometriosis, pelvic inflammatory disease) → Laparoscopy and dye
Laparoscopy is more invasive than HSG or HyCoSy – it requires general anaesthetic. This allows one-step diagnosis and treatment of conditions such as endometriosis and adhesions (scarring).

Figure 9.1 Fertility tests and investigations

sperm may be needed. IVF cannot compensate for age and declining egg quality so older women may be told that their best chance would be with donated eggs. Currently, about half of all live births in women over 40 are from donor eggs. If you are unable to carry a pregnancy for medical reasons, then surrogacy may be an option. The Human Fertilization and Embryology Association (HFEA) provides information on licensed fertility clinics and all aspects of assisted fertility.

Funding for NHS fertility treatment (including IVF) varies across the UK, with access dependent on your postcode and your personal circumstances. In England, the Local Clinical Commissioning Groups

(CCGs) make the decisions on who will qualify for funding. For more information on fairer access to NHS funding, see Fertility Network UK.

Miscarriage

Some women do get pregnant but the pregnancy fails – this is called a miscarriage and is very common. Around 10–20 pregnancies in every 100 (10–20 per cent) miscarry. This can happen to women of any age, but it is more common in older women due to chromosomal abnormalities with the pregnancy. If this happens to you, there is a high chance you will be able to have a successful pregnancy in the future. However, some women who miscarry repeatedly (three or more consecutive miscarriages) may require specialist help to diagnose any treatable causes. You can find out more information from your doctor, nurse or midwife, or by contacting the Miscarriage Association (see Resources).

If you are not getting pregnant or you conceive but miscarry, you may find the whole situation overwhelming. Many women (and men) who have fertility problems express feelings of anxiety, fear, frustration, anger, despair, loss of control, and a sense of failure. If you are struggling to cope with an uncertain future, ask your doctor whether you can see a counsellor within the practice, or contact a specialist fertility counsellor through the British Infertility Counselling Association (see Resources).

It is not within the scope of this book to address the physical or emotional aspects of miscarriage or infertility in any detail – whether you are struggling to conceive your first child or you already have a child, but are unable to complete your family. If you would like more in-depth information, see Further reading in the Resources.

Resources: Contact details and further reading

This section provides contact details for organizations that offer further information and advice on the topics discussed in this book.

Andrology Solutions www.andrologysolutions.co.uk Specialists in male fertility – provide kits for self-insemination.

Association of Chartered Physiotherapists in Women's Health (ACPWH) www.acpwh.org.uk Specialist Physiotherapists for women's health issues.

Breast Cancer Now www.breastcancernow.org UK-based breast cancer research and care charity.

British Acupuncture Council www.acupuncture.org.uk Maintains a register of accredited acupuncturists.

British Infertility Counselling Association (BICA) www.bica.net Provides a list of fertility counsellors to help you cope with the emotional aspects of infertility.

Brook www.brook.org.uk Confidential sexual health and wellbeing information and support for young people.

Cancer Screening Service www.cancerscreening.nhs.uk Cancer screening information in the UK.

College of Sexual and Relationship Therapists (COSRT) www.cosrt.org.uk Leading membership organization for therapists specializing in sexual and relationship issues.

Daisy Network www.daisynetwork.org Support and information for women who have a premature menopause.

Disability, Pregnancy and Parenthood www.disabledparent.org.uk Information on pre-pregnancy and pregnancy plus peer support for disabled parents.

Drinkaware www.drinkaware.co.uk Provides support lines and advice about reducing alcohol.

Drinkline www.nhs.uk/live-well/alcohol-advice Provides advice and support for reducing the amount of alcohol you drink.

Ectopic Pregnancy Trust www.ectopic.org.uk Support and information for women who have an ectopic pregnancy.

Faculty of Sexual and Reproductive Healthcare www.fsrh.org Information and guidance on contraception and sexual health.

Fertility Network UK www.fertilitynetworkuk.org Information and support for people coping with fertility delays.

Food Standards Agency www.food.gov.uk Guide to foods that you can trust – healthier, more sustainable choices.

Forward (Foundation of Woman's Health Research and Development) www.forwarduk.org.uk Information, research and policy about female genital mutilation.

Frank www.talktofrank.com Confidential drugs and alcohol information and where to go for help.

Health and Safety Executive www.hse.gov.uk Information and advice on health and safety at work.

Healthy Start www.healthystart.nhs.uk Information on healthy eating in pregnancy, breastfeeding and for families. Offers free vouchers which can be exchanged for vitamins, milk, fresh fruit and vegetables.

Human Fertilisation and Embryology Authority (HFEA) www.hfea.gov.uk Information on fertility clinics, assisted conception, services and publications.

Maternity Action www.maternityaction.org.uk Information on rights and benefits at work.

MHRA – Medicines and Healthcare products Regulatory Agency www.gov.uk/government/organisations/medicines-and-healthcare-products-regulatory-agency Regulates medicines, medical devices and blood components for transfusion in the UK.

Miscarriage Association www.miscarriageassociation.org.uk Help and support after miscarriage, ectopic pregnancy and molar pregnancy.

Money Matters www.direct.gov.uk Help and support about all money matters.

National Childbirth Trust (NCT) www.nct.org.uk Information on pregnancy, local antenatal classes, postnatal support groups, breastfeeding counsellors, workshops, baby and toddler groups.

National Travel Health Network (NaTHNaC) www.nathnac.net Provides up-to-date health information on international travel.

National Domestic Abuse Helpline (Refuge) www.nationaldahelpline.org.uk Information and support for anyone experiencing domestic abuse.

NHS Eatwell Guide www.nhs.uk/live-well/eat-well Information and guidance about eating a healthy balanced diet.

NHS website Health A–Z www.nhs.uk Information on all aspects of health, conditions, treatments, local services and healthy living. Look under 'W' for Women's Health.

NHS Smokefree www.nhs.uk/smokefree Information to help people stop smoking.

NHS Women's Health area www.nhs.uk/womens-health Information and support on health, wellbeing, conditions and screening.

NICE – The National Institute for Health and Care Excellence www.nice.org.uk Aims to improve outcomes for people using the NHS and other public and social care services. A major provider of clinical guidelines.

Relate www.relate.org.uk Offers relationship counselling for individuals and couples.

Royal College of Obstetricians and Gynaecologists www.rcog.org.uk Provides UK clinical guidelines and parallel patient information on reproductive health.

Tommy's www.tommys.org Information and publications on pre-pregnancy health, pregnancy, miscarriage and stillbirth. The site includes a Planning for Pregnancy Digital Tool. Tommy's Pregnancy Advice Line is a midwife-led service offering advice on planning pregnancy, pregnancy, problems, bereavement and emotional support after premature birth, miscarriage or stillbirth.

Verity www.verity-pcos.org.uk Information and support for women with polycystic ovary syndrome (PCOS).

Organizations teaching fertility awareness methods

The following organizations provide teaching in fertility awareness methods using a combination of indicators.

UK

FertilityUK provides evidence-guided information on fertility awareness methods and access to a network of accredited practitioners, some of whom work in the NHS and provide free instruction. FertilityUK is a secular (non-religious) organization. It provides training and updating for health professionals, but practitioners are responsible for their own practice and continuing professional development: www.fertilityuk.org

International

The following organizations provide access to fertility awareness teaching and resources: some are within health services but most are independent private services. Some groups have a religious orientation.

Australia: Australian Council of Natural Family Planning: www.acnfp.com.au
Canada: Serena provides access to teaching in English and French: www.serena.ca
Europe: European Institute for Family Life Education. A non-governmental organization with member associations all over Europe and beyond: www.ieef.eu
New Zealand: Natural Fertility New Zealand: www.naturalfertility.co.nz
USA: Association of Fertility Awareness Professionals provides access to a network of educators from a variety of backgrounds: www.fertilityawarenessprofessionals.com
Toni Weschler, *Taking Charge of your Fertility* book and app www.tcoyf.com/
Worldwide resources on Standard Days Method, TwoDay Method and Lactational Amenorrhoea Method: Institute for Reproductive Health Georgetown University: www.irh.org

Further reading

The Complete Guide to Fertility Awareness, **Jane Knight, Routledge, 2017.**
Written by a fertility nurse specialist (one of the authors), this book is aimed primarily at health professionals but it is easily readable by anyone wishing to deepen their understanding of fertility. It provides a comprehensive review of the history and development of fertility awareness methods and an in-depth look at the scientific background of the different fertility indicators and how they correlate. It includes self-assessment exercises, case studies on planning and avoiding pregnancy, and over 600 references to scientific papers.

The Fertility Book, **Adam Balen and Grace Dugdale, Vermillion, 2021.**
Written by a gynaecologist and nutrition scientist, this book provides comprehensive information on infertility investigations and treatments. It also addresses preconception health, diet and lifestyle.

Appendix: Blank charts and instructions for use

Blank chart for avoiding pregnancy

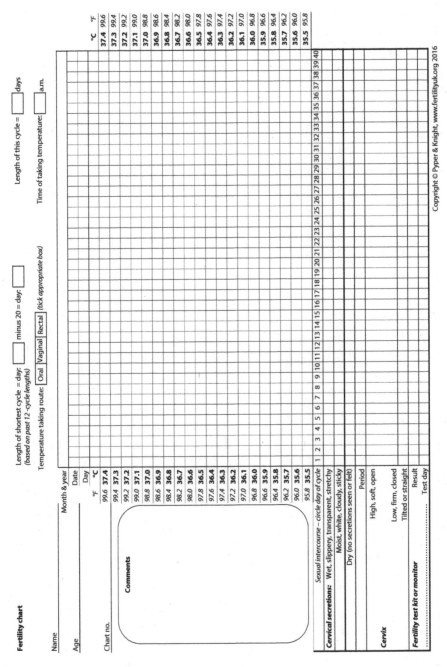

Instructions for use of the chart (avoiding pregnancy)

Instructions for use of the fertility chart

Temperature

1. Use a Celsius (centigrade) digital thermometer. Follow the manufacturer's instructions. Most digital thermometers have an audible bleep, a last memory recall feature and a low-battery warning indicator.

2. Take your temperature immediately on waking, before getting out of bed or doing anything. If recording time varies by more than 1 hour, note this on the chart.

3. Place the bulb of the thermometer under your tongue in contact with the floor of your mouth, close your lips gently and leave until the thermometer produces the audible bleep (takes about 1 minute). Oral temperatures are usually reliable, but if readings are erratic, your FA practitioner may suggest an internal reading – vaginal or rectal. Make any change in temperature-taking route at the beginning of the cycle.

4. Remove the thermometer, read it and mark it with a dot in the centre of the appropriate square, not on the line. Join the dots to form a continuous graph.

5. If you miss a day, leave a gap on the chart. (Do not join non-consecutive dots.)

6. Clean the thermometer with a little cotton wool and cold water.

Cycle length

1. The first day of your period is day 1 of the cycle. Start a new chart on that day.

2. If your period (fresh red bleed) starts during the day, transfer that morning's temperature to a new chart.

3. Record your cycle lengths to estimate the length of your shortest cycle.

Cervical secretions

1. Observe secretions throughout the day and record on the chart in the evening.

2. Observe the sensation (feel) and colour (look) and do the finger-test (touch).

3. Describe the secretions using shading in the appropriate box:
   - Period, including blood spotting
   - No secretions seen or felt (dry)
   - Moist, white or cloudy, sticky secretions·
   - Wet, slippery, transparent, stretchy secretions.

4. Indicate peak day by extending the shaded area in the column vertically upwards to correlate with the temperature readings.
   Peak day is the *last* day of highly fertile secretions (last day in top box). Peak day can only be recognized in retrospect (day after peak) when the secretions have changed back to show less fertile characteristics (marked in a lower box).

Cervix (optional)

The infertile cervix is represented by:
- a solid black circle showing it to be firm and closed: ●
- the circle is placed low down, showing it lower in the vagina
- a slanted line drawn below shows the tilt: /

The fertile cervix is represented by:
- an open circle showing softening: ○
- an inner circle showing that the cervix is more open: ◎
- the circle is placed higher, showing it higher in the vagina
- a vertical line below shows the cervix straight in position: I

Cyclical symptoms (optional)

- Indicate abdominal pain, breast or mood changes

Fertility monitoring devices (optional)

- Indicate test days and results.
- Correlate results with observed fertility indicators.

Sexual intercourse

- Indicate intercourse by circle around the appropriate day.
- If combing with barrier methods, indicate whether sex is protected or unprotected (e.g. C for condom)
- Note any other sexual activity such as withdrawal method which could result in pregnancy.

Comments

Note late nights, alcohol, illness, drugs, travel or stressful times on the appropriate days and/or in the comments box.

Further help: Contact FertilityUK at www.fertilityuk.org

Local FAM practitioner: Tel:_____

Blank chart for planning pregnancy with instructions for use

FERTILITY AWARENESS CHART: PLANNING PREGNANCY

Name: ....

Instructions for use:

- o Observe cervical secretions throughout the day. Record on the chart in the evening.
- o The first day of the period (fresh red bleed) is day 1 of the cycle. Start a new chart at the start of each period (four blank charts below)
- o Record days of period; dry days; moist, white, cloudy, sticky secretions; and days of wetter, slippery, transparent, stretchy secretions.
- o The fertile time starts at the first sign of any secretions and continues for three days after peak day (last day of wet, stretchy secretions).
- o Aim for sex at least two to three times per week. The days with wetter, transparent, stretchy secretions have the highest chance of pregnancy.

Example chart   Sept/Oct

Date	7	8	9	10	11	12	13	14	15	16	17	18	19	20	21	22	23	24	25	26	27	28	29	30	1	2	3
Day	W	T	F	S	S	M	T	W	T	F	S	S	M	T	W	T	F	S	S	M	T	W	T	F	S	S	M

Peak day →

Wet, slippery, transparent, stretchy — 1 2 3

Moist, white, cloudy, sticky

Dry (no secretions seen or felt)

Period

Day of cycle – circle intercourse: 1 2 3 4 5 6 ⑦ 8 ⑨ 10 ⑪ ⑫ ⑬ ⑭ 15 16 17 ⑱ 19 20 ㉑ 22 23 ㉔ 25 26 27 28 29 30 31 32 33 34 35 36 37 38 39 40

← Fertile Time →

Chart number:

| Date | | | | | | | | | | | | | | | | | | | | | | | | | | | | | | | | | | | | | | | | |

| Day | | | | | | | | | | | | | | | | | | | | | | | | | | | | | | | | | | | | | | | | |

Wet, slippery, transparent, stretchy

Moist, white, cloudy, sticky

Dry (no secretions seen or felt)

Period

Day of cycle – circle intercourse: 1 2 3 4 5 6 7 8 9 10 11 12 13 14 15 16 17 18 19 20 21 22 23 24 25 26 27 28 29 30 31 32 33 34 35 36 37 38 39 40

Chart number:

| Date | | | | | | | | | | | | | | | | | | | | | | | | | | | | | | | | | | | | | | | | |

| Day | | | | | | | | | | | | | | | | | | | | | | | | | | | | | | | | | | | | | | | | |

Wet, slippery, transparent, stretchy

Moist, white, cloudy, sticky

Dry (no secretions seen or felt)

Period

Day of cycle – circle intercourse: 1 2 3 4 5 6 7 8 9 10 11 12 13 14 15 16 17 18 19 20 21 22 23 24 25 26 27 28 29 30 31 32 33 34 35 36 37 38 39 40

Chart number:

| Date | | | | | | | | | | | | | | | | | | | | | | | | | | | | | | | | | | | | | | | | |

| Day | | | | | | | | | | | | | | | | | | | | | | | | | | | | | | | | | | | | | | | | |

Wet, slippery, transparent, stretchy

Moist, white, cloudy, sticky

Dry (no secretions seen or felt)

Period

Day of cycle – circle intercourse: 1 2 3 4 5 6 7 8 9 10 11 12 13 14 15 16 17 18 19 20 21 22 23 24 25 26 27 28 29 30 31 32 33 34 35 36 37 38 39 40

Chart number:

| Date | | | | | | | | | | | | | | | | | | | | | | | | | | | | | | | | | | | | | | | | |

| Day | | | | | | | | | | | | | | | | | | | | | | | | | | | | | | | | | | | | | | | | |

Wet, slippery, transparent, stretchy

Moist, white, cloudy, sticky

Dry (no secretions seen or felt)

Period

Day of cycle – circle intercourse: 1 2 3 4 5 6 7 8 9 10 11 12 13 14 15 16 17 18 19 20 21 22 23 24 25 26 27 28 29 30 31 32 33 34 35 36 37 38 39 40

Glossary/Useful words

Abstinence – Refraining from sexual intercourse and all genital contact.

Adenomyosis – A painful condition where endometrial tissue is found deep in the myometrium (muscle of the uterus).

Amenorrhoea – Absence of menstruation. Primary amenorrhoea is the complete absence of menstruation after puberty. Secondary amenorrhoea is the absence of menstruation for at least six months after having normal periods.

Anti-mullerian hormone (AMH) – A hormone produced by the ovaries which declines with age. A blood test for AMH gives some indication about a woman's ovarian (egg) reserve.

Antral follicles – Small resting follicles in the ovary. An internal scan can count the number of follicles to give an indication of a woman's ovarian reserve.

Basal body temperature (BBT) – The temperature of the body at rest, taken immediately on waking and before any activity – referred to here as the resting temperature. Ovulation causes a slight rise in resting temperature.

Biphasic chart – The two-phase temperature chart showing low-phase temperatures before ovulation followed by a rise of about 0.2 degrees Celsius (0.2 °C) around ovulation and remaining at the higher level until the next period starts.

Blastocyst – The stage about five to six days after fertilization when the early embryo has divided to form about 100 cells, which become the embryo and the placenta.

Body Mass Index (BMI) – A measure of a person's weight in relation to their height. This calculation is used to define normal weight, underweight, overweight and obesity.

Cervical ectropion – A harmless condition of the cervix in which the lining of the cervical canal protrudes onto the outer part of the cervix, resulting in increased cervical mucus secretion throughout the cycle and sometimes light bleeding.

Cervical secretions – Also known as vaginal secretions, this is the mucus from the cells lining the cervix. The quantity and quality vary with hormonal changes throughout the menstrual cycle.

Cervix – The lower part of the uterus that connects to the vagina. The cervical canal links the uterus to the vagina. It is lined with a mucus membrane, which produces cervical secretions. The opening of the cervix to the vagina is known as the external cervical os.

Chemical pregnancy (also known as biochemical pregnancy) – A very early miscarriage (up until five weeks of pregnancy). A home pregnancy test (or a blood test) detects hCG as the embryo starts to implant, but the pregnancy will not be detected by an ultrasound scan.

Clitoris – Sensitive organ found towards the front of the vulva which, when stimulated, can make a woman feel sexually aroused and can lead to orgasm. It is similar in origin to the male glans penis.

Conception – The process of getting pregnant that begins with fertilization of an egg by a sperm and ends with successful implantation of a fertilized egg in the endometrium.

Corpus luteum – The remains of the follicle after it has released an egg (also called the 'yellow body'). It produces progesterone in the second phase of the menstrual cycle (post-ovulatory) to help maintain a possible pregnancy.

Coverline – A technique used for identifying a rise in temperature associated with ovulation when using a fertility chart. A horizontal line is drawn on the line immediately above the highest of the low-phase temperatures. A cross is then drawn to divide the low- and high-phase temperatures.

Cystitis – Inflammation of the bladder and/or the urethra.

Ectopic pregnancy – A pregnancy that develops outside the uterus – usually in a fallopian tube. Although this is not common, it is very serious for the woman's health and usually requires emergency treatment. The pregnancy will be lost and the fallopian tube is damaged.

Egg – The mature female sex cell, which carries the woman's genetic contribution to her child (also referred to as the oocyte or the ovum).

Ejaculation – The release of seminal fluid (containing sperm) from the penis during male orgasm.

Embryo – The term used for a developing baby for the first eight weeks of pregnancy.

Endometriosis – A painful condition where the lining of the uterus (endometrium) starts to grow in other places, such as the ovaries, fallopian tubes OR in the pelvic area.

Endometrium – The lining of the uterus. This is shed about once a month as a period as part of the menstrual cycle. If conception occurs, the fertilized egg implants in the endometrium.

Epididymis – A network of coiled tubes at the top of the testicles where sperm gain their motility (ability to move) and their capacity to fertilize the egg.

Estrogen – A female sex hormone that is responsible for some changes that occur in the menstrual cycle. It also controls female characteristics such as breast growth, female body fat distribution and body shape. Synthetic estrogen is used in some forms of hormonal contraception.

Fallopian tubes – The small tubes linking the ovaries to the uterus. These are the tubes that are cut or blocked during female sterilization.

Fecundity – Being fertile.

Female genital mutilation (FGM) – The partial or total removal of a woman's external genitals or other deliberate injury to her genital organs. It is illegal in the UK.

Fertile time – The days of the menstrual cycle which include the day of ovulation, and the days before and after ovulation when intercourse may lead to pregnancy.

Fertility – The ability to reproduce.

Fertility awareness – An understanding of the pattern of fertility and infertility throughout the menstrual cycle and an appreciation of a woman's fertility potential at different stages of reproductive life.

Fertility awareness methods (FAMs) – This includes all family planning methods which are based on identifying the fertile time. Abstinence may be used during the fertile time (natural family planning) or FAMs may be combined with barrier methods.

Fertilization – The joining of a man's sperm with a woman's egg. This usually takes place in the outer third of the fallopian tube.

Fetus – The term used for a developing baby after the eighth week of pregnancy.

Fibroid – A non-cancerous growth that develops in or around the uterus. Sometimes called uterine myomas or leiomyomas.

Follicle – Small fluid-filled structure in the ovary which contains the egg.

Follicle-stimulating hormone (FSH) – A hormone produced by the pituitary gland to stimulate the production of follicles in the ovary.

Follicular phase – The time in the menstrual cycle from the start of the period until ovulation (pre-ovulation phase). This phase of the cycle varies in length.

Foreskin – The sleeve of skin that surrounds and protects the head of the penis.

Genes – The genetic material carried in chromosomes that determine a person's sex and characteristics.

Genetics – The science of the study of genes.

Gender – Gender refers to the characteristics of women, men, girls and boys that are socially constructed. This includes the behaviours and roles associated with being a woman, man, girl or boy, as well as their relationships with each other. Gender is different from sex, which refers to the different biological and physiological characteristics of women, men and intersex persons such as chromosomes, hormones and reproductive organs.

Gender identity – Refers to a person's deeply felt, internal and individual experience and their own internal sense of self as a man, woman, neither or both, which may or may not correspond to the person's physiology or designated sex at birth.

Glans (glans penis) – The bell-shaped head of the penis. This is normally covered by the foreskin.

Hormone – A chemical messenger that circulates in the bloodstream and regulates different activities in the body.

Human chorionic gonadotrophin (hCG) – The pregnancy hormone produced as a result of implantation. This is the hormone a pregnancy test looks for.

Hymen – Thin layer of soft skin that surrounds or partially covers the vaginal opening in prepubescent girls. This may still be present after puberty.

Hymenoplasty – A surgical intervention that involves reconstructing the hymen. Hymenoplasty and virginity testing are illegal in the UK.

Implantation – The process by which the fertilized egg embeds in the endometrium.

Indicators of fertility – The signs and symptoms which indicate a woman's fertility. The major indicators are cycle length, resting temperature, cervical secretions and cervical changes.

Infertile times – The two distinct phases of the menstrual cycle when a woman has a low chance of conception. The time after ovulation – the late infertile time (post-ovulatory) – is the most effective, whereas the time before ovulation – the early infertile time (preovulatory) – is only *relatively* infertile.

Infertility – Failure to conceive after regular unprotected vaginal intercourse for more than one year.

Labia – The inner and outer vaginal lips.

Luteal phase – The time in the menstrual cycle from ovulation to the next period (post-ovulatory phase). This phase has a fixed length of 10–16 days.

Luteinizing hormone (LH) – A hormone produced by the pituitary gland to trigger ovulation and stimulate the formation of the corpus luteum and the production of progesterone.

Menarche – This is the first menstrual period a girl experiences, usually this is around 11–13 years, but it may be earlier or later.

Menopause – The time in a woman's life when the ovaries stop producing eggs and her periods stop. She is no longer fertile. Menopause literally means 'end of menstruation' (final period).

Menstrual cycle (fertility cycle) – The sequence of changes in the ovaries and endometrium. This is under the control of the female sex hormones. The menstrual cycle lasts from the first day of the period, up to the day *before* the next period starts.

Menstruation – The monthly shedding of the endometrium, also known as a period.

Miscarriage – The unplanned loss of a pregnancy before 24 completed weeks.

Molar pregnancy – A rare condition where the placenta overgrows and the embryo does not form correctly.

Monophasic chart – A temperature chart which does not show the typical biphasic pattern. The temperatures remain on one level, suggesting that ovulation did not occur.

Orchitis – Inflammation of the testicle(s) from a urinary infection, sexually transmitted infection or as a complication of mumps.

Orgasm – Climax of sexual excitement in the male or female. Ejaculation usually accompanies male orgasm. Female orgasm is more varied depending on physical and psychological factors.

Ovarian (egg) reserve – The approximate number of eggs a woman has left. A woman's age combined with her ovarian reserve predict how well her ovaries would respond to IVF treatment.

Ovary – Small organs on either side of the uterus that produce ova (eggs) in structures called follicles. Ovaries also produce the female sex hormones – estrogen and progesterone.

Ovulation – The release of a mature egg from one of the ovaries each menstrual cycle.

Ovum (plural **ova**, also known as **oocytes**) – The mature egg produced by the ovary.

Peak day – The *last* day of the wet, transparent stretchy secretions. (It can only be recognized retrospectively.) Peak day correlates closely with ovulation.

Penis – The male reproductive organ outside the body responsible for ejaculating seminal fluid.

Perimenopause – The time leading up to the menopause when periods stop.

Period – *See:* Menstruation.

Pituitary gland – Small gland at the base of the brain that produces a number of hormones, including hormones controlling the function of the ovaries and testes.

Placenta – Roundish, flat, spongy organ that connects the embryo/fetus to the pregnant woman via the umbilical cord. It is responsible for transferring nourishment from the woman to the fetus and removal of the fetus's waste products. After delivery, this becomes part of the afterbirth.

Pre-ejaculatory fluid – The small amount of lubricating fluid which is released involuntarily from a man's penis during sexual excitement prior to ejaculation. This fluid may contain sperm.

Pregnancy – The condition of nurturing the unborn embryo or fetus from conception to birth. A pregnancy lasts around 280 days (40 weeks) and is calculated from the first day of the last period.

Progesterone – A female sex hormone that is responsible for some changes that occur in the menstrual cycle. It also is important in maintaining normal pregnancy.

Progestogen – A synthetic form of progesterone, found in hormonal methods of contraception.

Prostate – A gland situated at the base of the male bladder. Its nutritive secretions add volume to make up the seminal fluid.

Prostatitis – Inflammation of the prostate gland.

Scrotum – The soft pouch of skin that holds and protects a man's testicles. It is responsible for regulating the temperature of the testicles to optimize sperm production.

Seminal fluid (semen) – Creamy-white viscous fluid ejaculated from the penis at orgasm. It contains sperm and secretions from the prostate and seminal vesicles.

Seminal vesicles – A pair of glands which open into the top of the male urethra. Secretions from the seminal vesicles contribute to the seminal fluid.

Sperm –The male sex cell made in the testicles which carries the man's genetic contribution to his child.

Stillbirth – When a baby is born dead after the twenty-fourth week of pregnancy.

Subfertility – Reduced fertility with a prolonged time to achieve pregnancy.

Temperature *See:* Basal body temperature.

Temperature rise – The shift in resting temperature (of around 0.2 °C) which divides the low-phase temperatures from the high-phase temperatures on a biphasic chart.

Temperature spike – A single temperature recording which is 0.2 °C or more above the one on both sides. This may be caused by a disturbance such as drinking alcohol.

Testicle – Men have two testicles or testes contained in the scrotum. They produce sperm and the hormone testosterone.

Testosterone – A male sex hormone that is responsible for sperm production and for male sexual characteristics.

Urinate – To pass urine through the urethra.

Urethra – Tube that carries urine from the bladder to the urinary opening. In men, the urethra also carries the seminal fluid.

Uterus – Also called the womb. This is where an embryo/fetus develops when a woman becomes pregnant.

Vagina – A muscular tube about 7–10 cm long that connects the cervix to the vulva.

Vas deferens – Tube that carries sperm from the testicles to the penis. This is the tube that is cut during male sterilization (vasectomy).

Vulva – The female genitals outside the body. It includes the entrance to the vagina, the urethra, the labia and the clitoris.

Index

abdominal bloating, 56
abortion, effect on future conception, 156
abstinence, 2, 5, 80–81
abusive relationships, 117
acupuncture, 154
adenomyosis, 57
adhesions, 164, 165
age, and decline in fertility, 10, 160–1
air travel, 145–6
alcohol, 140–2
allergies, 136
amenorrhoea, 175
  lactational (see lactational amenorrhoea method) 90–3
antibiotics, 13
antihistamines, 62
anti-mullerian hormone (AMH), 163
antral follicle count (AFC), 163–4
apps, 64–5
arousal fluid,13, 61
assisted conception, 27, 153–4

bacterial vaginosis (BV), 123, 124
barrier methods, 2, 81
Bartholin's glands, 13
basal body temperature (BBT), 20
Basic Infertile Pattern (BIP), 93–5, 96–100
beta-carotene 121
biphasic charts, 45–6, 104
bleeding after childbirth, 92
bleeding during perimenopause, 105–6
bleeding between periods, 57
bloating, 56
blood tests, 162–3
body mass index (BMI), 129
bottle feeding, 89, 101
breastfeeding, 4, 89–100, 157
breasts, 13–14
  changes in, 14, 57

caffeine, 137
cervical ectropion 60
cervical screening, 124–5
cervical secretions, 11–12, 17, 18, 32–3
  changes during menstrual cycle, 34–9
  difficulties with monitoring, 60–2
  monitoring, 35–9, 51–2
  in perimenopause, 104–5
  variations after hormonal contraception, 84
cervix, 11–12, 17, 18
  changes after childbirth, 53, 94
  monitoring changes, 52–6
childbirth
  cervical changes, 53
  conception after, 157–8
chromosomes, 114–15, 161
Clearblue fertility monitor, 63
clitoris, 7, 29
complementary therapies, 154
conception, 25–6
  assisted, 27, 153–4
  delays to, 156–66
  preparation for, 115–55
  process, 27–8
  and sexual intercourse, 28
  and temperature changes, 48–9
contraception
  after childbirth if not breastfeeding, 101
  barrier methods, 2, 81
  breastfeeding as, 89–93
  fertility monitors, 63–4
  hormonal, 82
  natural family planning (NFP), 2, 80–1
  stopping, 127, 156
  using fertility awareness methods (FAMs), 66–81
  and weight concerns, 131–2